MASTERING HEALTHY AGING FOR MEN

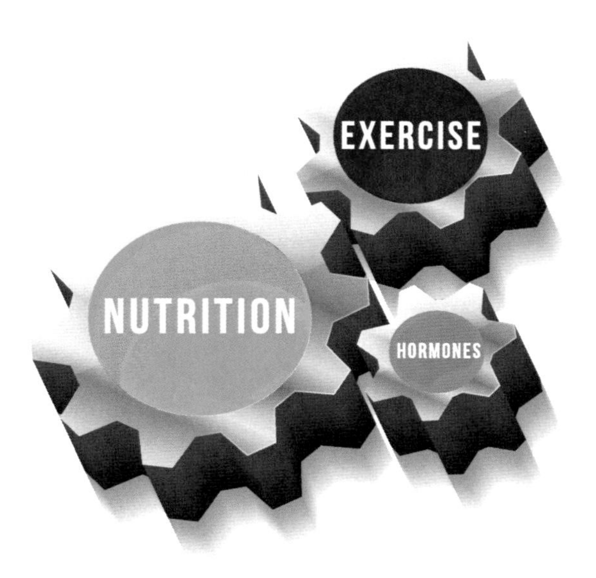

NUTRITION, EXERCISE *and* HORMONE REPLACEMENT THERAPY

TODD DAVID GREENBERG M.D., CSCS,*D *and* JEFFREY PARK LEAKE M.D., CPT

Cover Design: Kristi Eakin
Editors: Laurel Avery, Roland Combes, and Juliette Siegfried
at ServingMed.com
Contributing Editor: Noah Greenberg
Graphics & Citations: Natalie Vorobyova

ISBN-13: 978-1511642361
ISBN-10: 151164236X

Copies of this book and other informative volumes in the series can be obtained from the website www.benevitahealth.com.

To my mother and father, who left us far too early in life.

TDG

Acknowledgments

We would like to thank Bonnie Paur for collaboration on Nutritional Concepts; Robert Willix, MD, for his support in developing the training course; the Partners and Fellows at Cenegenics Elite Health; Beth Traylor, MD, and the Cenegenics Education and Research Foundation; and all the physicians who have completed training and certification. We are also are indebted to Kari Lennartson for collaboration on Exercise Concepts; Natalie Vorobyova for meticulous citation documentation and graphic creation; Kristi Eakin for the cover design and publishing assistance; Nancy Gerth for the extensive indexing; and Laurel Avery and Juliette Siegfried at ServingMed.com for their patient and thorough medical editing, book layout, and typesetting.

Finally, for their support throughout the writing of this book, Dr. Greenberg would like to thank his mentors, friends, and family; and Dr. Leake would like to thank his wife Amy.

TABLE OF CONTENTS

ABBREVIATIONS AND DEFINITIONS

TG: triglycerides

DMII: diabetes type II (poor diet leading to acquired diabetes)

CVD: cardiovascular disease

GL: glycemic load

GI: glycemic index

Endothelium: blood vessel lining

PUFA: polyunsaturated fatty acid (e.g. omega-3 and omega-6 fatty acids)

MUFA: monounsaturated fatty acid (e.g. fatty acids found in olive oil)

EFA: Essential fatty acid—a form of unsaturated fatty acid. The body cannot make EFAs so they must be consumed directly.

ALA: alpha linolenic acid—an omega-3 fatty acid

LA: linoleic acid—an omega-6 fatty acid

Primary prevention: Doing something to prevent the likelihood of developing a disease or condition, such as taking aspirin to reduce risk of heart attack.

Hedonics: the study of the how pleasure influences the choices we make. In this text it refers to how the unchecked desire to eat something tasty leads to obesity.

Catechins: A type of flavonoid that is a type of antioxidant.

Endothelial health: health of the blood vessel lining. When inflammation from poor lifestyle choices like smoking damages the lining, higher rates of heart attacks occur.

HIIT: short-duration high-intensity interval training—prescribed from your measured heart rate max (not estimated). Optimal 4 times a week to make heart health gains, 3 times a week for maintenance.

LSD: long slow distance. Helpful to increase heart health, but once a week is sufficient (5 mile run).

1RM: maximum weight you can lift with that particular exercise. It is the 1 rep max, and measures maximum single effort strength. A 15RM weight would measure your endurance strength.

SAID: specific adaptations to imposed demand—a guiding principle of training that says basically, "compete like you train, train like you compete."

GAS: general adaptation syndrome—a training athlete's response to training. Your body first responds with alarm, then resistance, then exhaustion.

Concurrent training: doing both HIIT and weight training weekly. If performed on the same day, do weights first.

CHAPTER I

NUTRITION

"Motivation is what gets you started. Habit is what keeps you going."

Jim Ryun

Introduction to Nutrition

*T*his chapter has been designed to help individuals better understand food and use that knowledge to improve their health.

We will reframe how you view food and its components and how they affect the buildup of body fat. You will become familiar with body fat and how it is an unhealthy generator of inflammation that taxes the rest of your systems. We will show you why foods that increase your insulin levels (e.g., high GL foods) stop you from losing weight. Such foods keep you fat by preventing you from using fat as fuel, the alternative energy source in your body. We will show you why body fat leads to low quality life and premature death, from a scientific perspective.

We explain appetite— how it works biologically, and how the biggest problem in managing weight has less to do with biology and more to do with the overabundance of food, low quality food products, and how we respond to our environment.

We show you why some diet plans work and others don't— and why it makes no difference in the long run.

We provide a number of answers to commonly asked questions. But if your questions are not answered in the book, please e-mail us at info@benevitahealth.com. We want to accurately answer those questions.

Most importantly, we provide you with a foundation for entering a ew stage of life that will allow you to enjoy food, but know whether it s promoting your health or detracting from it. After all, it is your life, nd you have a right to enjoy it. Our job is to give you the knowledge o understand when enjoying it is promoting a higher quality of life nd longevity.

A side note:

Many compassionate and intelligent care providers have concluded "will power" is not central to the solution of the epidemic of obesity; here we differ. We show you why, biologically, it is the only answer to the epidemic of obesity, short of controlling food access.

We are genetically programmed (some more efficiently than others) to store available calories in the event of a lack of available calories, such as during a famine. When food is available, it is perfectly natural to eat. It is what has contributed to survival over the millennia, until very recently. Such behavior is now contributing to earlier death, rather than longer life. Over time, but far beyond our lifetime, we will probably see genetic pressure toward improved survival of those who resist stuffing their faces every time food is presented. We are in transition, evolutionarily speaking.

Because the obese are metabolically altered by poor nutrition, with chronic inflammation and hormonal imbalances, the challenges of managing their body fat reduction are greater. Medications and/or surgery can be helpful to get them to healthy body fat levels. However, no matter how the weight loss was achieved, to maintain those healthy levels everyone inevitably requires a component of restraint and needs to reshape how food is perceived. Self-discipline is required in the reshaping because of the ubiquitous nature of food, especially highly palatable, energy-dense (while being nutrient-poor) processed foods. We show you how your wonderful brain is equipped to restrain primitive impulses. Plus, isn't it empowering take charge of your actions?

We recognize the central role of hedonics (liking and wanting) in appetite regulation, and recognize that desiring a food product can be similar to desiring a drug, though there are fundamental differences. **We commonly accept that it is best to refrain from many impulses in life; impulses that would get us into social trouble. But for some reason we think refraining from eating impulses does not need similar effort. It does.** Not surprisingly, we now know we *can* learn to like foods such as spinach, kale, and broccoli. MRI studies show it.

Thus, we compassionately disagree with those who say that body fat loss is not within the sphere of the patient's control. It must be.

Understanding Nutrition

Part I

*N*utrition is the cornerstone of aging well. Middle age is when we often start noticing the impact of our nutritional (and non-nutritional) choices over the past decades. Although it plays a crucial role in how we age, genetics is not yet a factor we can change. Exciting research is being conducted in epigenetics, which describes the effect of the environment on gene activity, but the field is still in its infancy. There are numerous daily life activities that affect whether certain genes are "turned on"—ones involving nutrition, sleep, exercise, and stress.

There is research that points to the possibility of indirect control of genetics through environmental factors, such as nutrition. Once reliable testing methods have been made available, with results that can be implemented into a workable program, we will use them to help you and others.

This book focuses on what measures we can change today to improve how we age. Nutrition, while a lifetime investment, is the single most powerful tool we have to improve our aging process at any stage of life.

You as a Banker

Conceptually, we view the assets of nutrition, exercise, sleep, and hormone optimization as a type of currency or investment towards the later years of life. The most important bank for building a longer life is the *Heart Bank*. Although the Heart Bank does improve longevity, it also contributes to the enjoyment of those years more fully, more youthfully. Other banks you can add to promote living young include your *Bone Bank*, *Muscle Bank*, and *Brain Bank*. The Bone and Muscle

Banks are easily the most important to help keep you independent and out of a nursing home. Although that might have been less of an issue in decades past because our lifespan was shorter, in the coming decades, increasing numbers of frail people will require assisted living. Frailty is a direct consequence of poorly developed Bone and Muscle Banks. Finally, we know the least about how to build the Brain Bank, but we are working on it vigorously. Maxing out your contributions to the other banks certainly has synergistic effects for the Brain Bank as well.

Finally, remember that where you have assets you also have liabilities. The two biggest liabilities against building your banks are Aging and Inflammation.

More liability limits your capacity to repair. Unfortunately, most of us literally and conceptually, have way too many liabilities. Like our understanding of the Brain Bank, we are still in the early stages of understanding how inflammation contribute broadly to our liabilities. We know it is central to development of plaque and therefore cardiovascular disease, and that poor sleep contributes to inflammation. Conceptually, we view sleep as reparative on a cellular level. Without that time to repair, maintaining the "systems" of a slowly degenerating body becomes impossible, no matter how strong the will and drive. Cells need time to recover from oxidative stresses, especially in a world that exposes us to more environmental insults than ever before. Poor sleep quality and low sleep quantity are known to contribute to excess inflammation. Inflammation is your body's response to a broad range of irritants, whether they are toxic food products, lack of sleep, stress, or carrying too much body fat.

Inflammation contributes substantially to a shorter life span (for example, from heart disease) and a lower quality of life (due to chronic disease).

Aging is inevitable; a liability that must be taken on regardless of what you do. Minimizing other liabilities and maximizing your Banks' assets are the best ways to mitigate against aging. Later in the book we discuss how maintaining optimal hormone systems, despite aging, allows you to maximize your assets and minimize your liabilities.

The better you build your banks, the better you can manage the liabilities that come with poor sleep and inflammation, to a degree. As you read these chapters, keep in mind the four banks you will be aiming to build and how you can keep in check the liability of inflammation.

It is important to note that your balance of assets and liabilities is affected by genetics. Think of inheriting "good genes" as something of a trust fund. Genetics are pretty much fixed at this point in the game—good or bad. You can affect, to a small degree, which genes are turned on by what you do with lifestyle factors, such as nutrition and exercise. Currently, we know only a fraction of how genes really contribute to your long-term health and aging, and even less about what to do with that information.

For now, it is in your best interest to focus on what you *can* change. The areas you can change that will have the most dramatic impact on your life include nutrition, exercise, sleep, and when it is time, consider hormone replacement therapy to optimize your body's receptiveness to those lifestyle changes and reduce your overall rate of decay. It is all downhill after 30; it is just a matter of how fast you slide.

The Leake-Greenberg Window of Opportunity

It's all about the health of your blood vessels

Before reading further, we want to share with you a principle we have found very useful in understanding who will benefit the most from our preventive approach to aging well. This principle will become especially important when considering hormone optimization therapy. We believe everyone benefits from improved nutrition and exercise, but there is an ideal window, after which their efforts will result in less protective and preventive benefits. Unfortunately for a few, the consequences of decades of poor choices in the areas of nutrition and exercise/sleep, are unveiled during middle age. The reparative and sustaining hormonal systems begin to decline faster than during the years before middle age, and thus the impact of poor choices becomes more evident. Beginning hormone replacement after this ideal window might incur increased risk for both men and women, depending on the underlying damage—particularly damage to your blood vessels and cardiovascular system. For this reason, we developed the guideline that reminds us and other clinicians that it is not age that determines the safety of intense lifestyle changes and hormone therapy. It is the person's underlying vascular health. Our textbook explains more in depth about the *Leake-Greenberg (LG) Window of Opportunity*, summarized here:

The *LG Window of Opportunity* is a broadly applicable concept that states,

"Patients who are not burdened by significant inflammation-induced disorders such as endothelial dysfunction or hormone-resistant states are ideal candidates for primary prevention therapies, such as nutrition, exercise, and hormone optimizing."

Following is the specific application of *LG Window of Opportunity* to the area of nutrition:

- In terms of nutrition, the *Leake-Greenberg Window of Opportunity* occurs before hormone-resistant states (insulin/incretin/leptin) become irreversible. These thresholds are still being developed. Regarding insulin resistance: by the time a patient requires subcutaneous insulin injections, it is unlikely the resistant state will be reversible, although it can be managed and improved.

Primary disease prevention means that "I don't have a disease, and if I perform this intervention (take a pill, exercise) I won't ever develop the disease." Secondary disease prevention means "I have this disease, and if I perform this intervention, it won't get worse."

One of the problems with our current public health approach to preventive medicine is that *testing is not prevention.* It is just testing. Unfortunately, this is where the academic, ivory tower physicians miss the boat. While testing certainly has its place, if I run a test and find a disease is present, I haven't prevented anything. Prevention comes through sound nutrition and exercise. The good news is that these domains are entirely under your control, and cost virtually nothing.

We believe the insulin surges that cause endothelial damage are at the core of premature heart disease and a wide range of other disorders. There are three additional effects from insulin surges that cause sustained inflammation because they prevent you from using fat as fuel. Insulin surges cause fat creation (lipogenesis); they prevent fat breakdown (lipolysis); and they inhibit fat from being used as fuel (fatty acid β oxidation). High insulin levels keep you fat. Fat and insulin promote inflammation, which is directly associated with obesity. Inflammation is reduced with good nutrition, exercise, and hormone optimization—the triad of a sound aging program.

Disregard any bad choices made in the past.

We strive for everyone to find the sweet spot where their efforts are significant enough to yield the gains they are looking for, without being so difficult that they give up on the program. The changes we hope to help you make are lifelong changes, not short-term and fleeting gains. The most constructive way to approach finding your sweet spot is to make the best choices today that you can make, even if past decisions have not been the best. By approaching your decision-making in this way each day, you are more likely to make, on the whole, higher quality choices more frequently than lower quality ones.

Obesity

Part II

Obesity is arguably the single worst result of poor nutrition.

It is entirely preventable, but now surpasses cigarette smoking as the most costly preventable disease. The trend is unrelenting, and middle age is the peak of it all, though people are achieving the status of "obese" earlier and earlier, despite the fact the government actually redefined obesity to make it harder to qualify as "obese."

> ***Inflammation and poor cardiovascular health are direct consequences of obesity.***

Before we dive too deeply into obesity, we must clarify general concepts around the word "calorie." After all, it is excess calories that ultimately lead to obesity. However, placing too much importance on calories can also become an obstacle to executing a sound nutritional program. There is more to food and its impact on your body than the calorie count.

Obesity is the first step in a series of conditions that lead to premature death, as illustrated by Figure 2.1 on the following page:

Figure 2.1

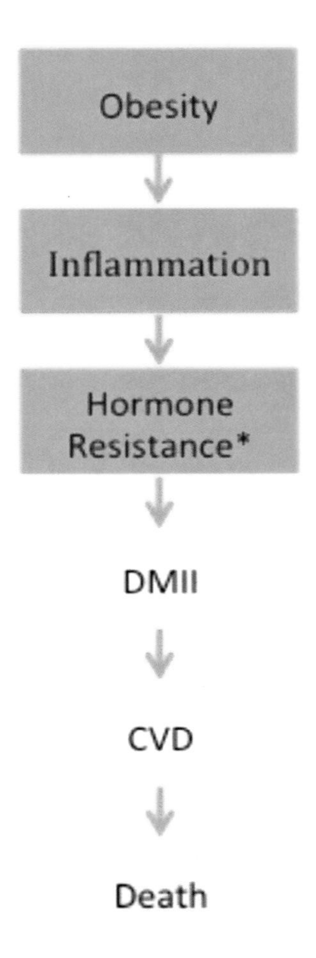

*insulin, incretin, leptin

A Calorie is Just a Calorie—Or is It?

A molecule that accounts for a calorie is both an energy source and a messenger.

Misconceptions about nutrition are common, including the idea that calorie counting is useful beyond the initial stages of a new nutritional program. Your body does a pretty good job on its own of keeping track of calories, and adjusts your food intake accordingly. Understand how many calories are packed into processed foods, how few calories there are in vegetables, and the rest are simple estimations. More important is to develop an understanding of what that calorie is doing to your insulin levels. We talk about that later when we explain glycemic index (GI) and glycemic load (GL). Even then, rather than calculating the GL, we want you be able to simply recognize when something is high or low GL. That's it as far as counting.

However, it is important to note that there are certain hard facts about energy balance that are always taking place, which we must be aware of. As applied to nutrition, the Law of Conservation states that

$$ES = EI - EO$$

*Where **ES** is stored energy (fat storage), **EI** is energy intake (calories from food) and **EO** is energy output (heat loss, exercise, and cooling from evaporation).*

When intake exceeds output, energy storage is positive. The energy can be stored as fat or muscle. When we are growing, we are in positive energy balance and we do not necessarily get fat. However, in adulthood, when energy storage is positive, it is most commonly stored as increased fat. This means in order to lose fat, we must be in a state of negative energy balance. As applied to the law of thermodynamics discussed above, it does not matter what form the calorie comes in because a calorie is just a unit of measure, like an inch or a foot. Thus, "a calorie is a calorie is a calorie" from the standpoint of thermodynamics. However, from another standpoint, "a calorie is not just a calorie".

The wide variety of fats, proteins, and carbohydrates play two roles. They serve as a source of energy (calories) and—less well understood—those macronutrient molecules also *serve as messengers that signal the digestive system and brain how to respond to the food eaten.*

> ***Food is both a source of calories and a way to send messages to the brain, regulating appetite and metabolism.***

Food is not just about energy intake. And, believe it or not, you are what you eat. More precisely, you are what your body *does* with what you eat (and what *it* ate or was fed).

This is important, because it illustrates a common problem in nutrition. Although it can be useful to focus on a particular aspect of nutrition, such as energy balance and thermodynamics, one must always step back and assess what that means in the larger context of other important factors such as hormonal response, epigenetics, and hedonics. This is something that has not been accomplished very well by the many "experts" in the field, and accounts for the mass confusion among the public regarding nutritional science.

Context is always important. This is why the nutritional prescription is always based on an individual *needs analysis* that incorporates all the relevant factors and why "one size does not fit all."

Etiologies of Obesity

Myth: Obesity is caused by a more sedentary lifestyle and lack of physical work during the workday.

Truth: Obesity is a result of eating too much. How to refrain from eating too much is the challenge.

There are two main camps that claim different reasons for the global (not just the American) epidemic of obesity. One thought is that we move less, but eat the same as we did a century ago. We agree that we have clearly shifted our energy expenditure from more constant hourly work to more episodic leisure/exercise related activities. Our research suggests there has not been a substantial shift in total energy expenditure, though we do recognize there has been a consolidation of it—the gym workout, the ski weekend. In short, we do not believe reduced energy expenditure is a significant contributor to the global epidemic of obesity.

Observing the exercise industry's explosion parallel the explosion of obesity supports this conclusion. There is also sound data that suggest our bodies want to stay at the same weight, and adjusts food intake over time to maintain that weight. One factor that might be throwing a monkey wrench into that tendency more directly relates to food quality. We tend to maintain the same weight over time. We do so by eating similar weight and/or volumes of food each week. However, because processed foods are abnormally calorie-laden, that similar weight and volume of food results in a constant insult to the body in the form of inflammation and insulin surges. Excess calories, particularly from carbohydrates (carbs), build inflammatory fat tissue that sends signals via insulin that damages blood vessels and elevates triglycerides (TGs).

Thus, we believe the constant availability of food and the diminished quality of food products has been a more substantial contributor to obesity than reduced energy expenditure.

What leads to obesity?

Too much pleasure or indulgence with your food intake.

Processed Foods

- *Processed foods range from unhealthy to very unhealthy. Restaurants, frozen foods, and pseudo-meats are among the most unhealthy.*
- *Processed foods are best characterized as excessively palatable, energy dense, but nutrient poor.*

Processed foods cause inflammation

The Nurses' Health Study (NHS) shows a diet high in processed foods (soft drinks, refined grains, processed meats) is associated with inflammation. The same study showed a "prudent" diet including low-fat dairy products reduced inflammation, as did a study of the Mediterranean diet, which is high in fish, vegetables, and olive oil. The fruit, vegetable, lean meat, and dairy-rich DASH diet also showed reduced inflammation.

> ***Staying away from processed foods makes eating simple on many levels. For example, all the chemicals that are added to foods that are categorized as generally recognized as safe (GRAS) by the FDA, are not so safe.***

A few very common additives include the following:

- Sodium nitrate is a preservative used to add color and flavor to bacon, ham, hot dogs, lunch meats, smoked fish, and corned beef (essentially, processed meats). It is also used to kill rodents. In natural products, such as vegetables, it is probably a healthy source of nitric oxide formation, dilating blood vessels. It also has anti-microbial action. It is highly debated whether or not the added nitrates are why processed meats are bad for you. What is not debated is that processed meats lead to an earlier death. We recommend you minimize added sodium nitrates in your diet and leave the fine points of biochemistry to the scientists.
- BHA (butylated hydroxyanisole) and BHT (butylated hydrozyttoluene) are also preservatives; they are petroleum-derived and act as both antioxidants and oxidizing agents. Oxidation damages our cells' DNA and promotes cancer. As would be expected, the data is quite controversial as to whether the net effect of preservatives justifies the benefits. We do not recommend them. Preservatives are not to your benefit, but to the benefit of the manufacturer's bottom line because they allow foods to stay on the shelves longer. If the food is unattractive or spoiled you probably aren't going to buy it. Preservatives are found in a wide range of products, including cereals, chewing gum, potato chips, and vegetable oils.

- Propyl gallate is a preservative often used with BHA and BHT, and is frequently found in meats, chicken soup, and chewing gum, for example. It is also an oxidant.
- Monosodium glutamate is a flavor enhancer used in soups, salads, chips, frozen entrées, and restaurant food. It causes headaches, nausea, and neurotoxicity.
- Food colorings are carcinogenic. Blue 1 and 2, Red 3, Green 3, and Yellow 6 have been studied most thoroughly and have been shown to be carcinogenic in mice. Blues are common in beverages, candy, baked goods, and pet food. Red is frequently found in dyed cherries, fruit cocktail, candy, and baked goods, and is associated with increased thyroid neoplasms. Green is found in candy and beverages, and is associated with increased bladder cancer. Yellow 6 is used in similar food products as above, but can also be found in gelatin. It is associated with renal and adrenal neoplasms.
- Olestra is an engineered fat that not only causes diarrhea, but directly impairs absorption of healthful foods, including carotenoids.

How Can Improved Nutrition Reduce Obesity?

Reduce insulin surges to burn fat instead of build fat

Basic Principles of minimizing fat building

1. Eat low-GL foods to keep insulin low
2. Have a moderate (25% of calories) high-quality protein intake
3. Eat whole food sources of omega-3 fats

Combating obesity through food planning strategically focuses on reducing food intake as well as correcting the mix of fat, protein, and carbohydrates (quantity and quality).

We focus on reducing the sugar/carb intake that causes insulin surges (high GL), and on increasing levels of high-quality protein daily. High quality protein comes largely from wild lean meats and coldwater fish such as salmon, halibut, cod, dover sole, and sablefish. Below we explain why.

Fat is not a macronutrient to monitor except knowing to avoid trans-fats (entirely) and keep saturated fats (largely from animals) to less than 7% of calories. In the context of a low-GL diet, one only needs to maximize the quality of the fat ingested (omega-3) and avoid disturbing the energy balance because fat, healthy or not, is energy-dense.

The GI and GL of carbohydrates play a critical role in heart disease risk factors, blood sugar control in people with type 2 diabetes mellitus (DMII), and in appetite control. GI and GL are important concepts for you to thoroughly understand. They will help you to know when you are eating healthy or unhealthy food. We discuss this in depth soon.

Meals containing high-quality protein have been shown to lengthen the time period until you are hungry again by causing increased satiety—the feeling of fullness—and increasing heat production. High-quality protein makes you feel fuller longer and burn more calories because making sugar (glucose) from protein takes a lot more energy than directly eating sugar or having the liver make it. Diets high in protein produce better weight control and weight loss than diets in which the protein is replaced by carbohydrate. High-protein diets are challenging the current recommendations of macronutrient mix and what we thought were the upper limits of protein intake. The Institute of Medicine changed its recommendations because evidence indicates we can and should be eating more high-quality protein, daily. They changed the acceptable daily protein intake for adults to 10%–35% of caloric intake, and for children (aged 4-18) 10%-30%. Other agencies will soon follow.

A diet with high protein intake also enhances body fat loss with preferential fat loss from visceral adipose tissue (VAT). Visceral adipose tissue is fat you often do not see, which is mixed with organs in your mid-section. It is that dangerous "belly fat" strongly associated with even more heart disease risk than subcutaneous fat, which tends to gather around the hips and thighs. Keep an eye out for new articles on more strategies and therapies that target visceral fat. They are coming.

Studies are mixed about the possible adverse effects of high-protein diets (35%) on renal function in healthy individuals, but our experience and quality evidence does not support a risk in patients with normal renal function. If you do not have bad kidneys (your doctor will tell you), you can be assured that a 35% protein diet is not harmful.

We encourage patients to focus on nutritional density when they are estimating the value of what they eat. Over time, we have found nutritionally dense foods contain many elements essential to good health that your multivitamin might not contain.

We have often observed an inverse relationship between nutritionally dense foods and energy-dense foods. You want to eat foods with high nutritional value, not just calories.

Finally, nutritionally rich foods often contain far more fiber than energy-dense foods. Fiber may be considered the fourth macronutrient, but that topic is complex. As you can guess, not all fiber is the same. For now, we will leave you with two important points to keep in mind about fiber:

- Carbs from high-fiber sources are do not elicit a strong insulin response
- Aim for 20-40 grams of natural source fiber daily.

Measuring Obesity

Measuring body fat is best done with DXA scanning.

There are several ways to measure fat in the body. Most studies you will read about use a technique called body mass index (BMI), which is cost-effective and adequate for most large population-based studies. BMI is defined as your weight divided by your height, squared; (kg/m^2). People with a high BMI tend to carry more fat. However, many very healthy athletic patients have a high BMI because they carry substantial lean tissue (bone, muscle, tendon, and water).

BMI ≥ 30 is considered obese
BMI ≥ 25 is considered overweight

If you are athletic with plenty of muscle, you should disrega BMI measurements. Conversely, many people with normal BMI ha obesity-related metabolic disease (they are “skinny fat”). Because these factors, the most recent 2013 guidelines from the American Soci of Bariatric Physicians (ASBP), an American Medical Associati (AMA) specialty board, used percent body fat >25% for men and >32 for women to define obesity. Using these more accurate definitio many “normal” people have been reclassified as overweight or obe You will want to assess body fat by either calipers in experienc hands (a collegiate trainer, for example) or have a dual-energy X-r absorptiometry (DXA) scan performed by a team like BeneVita Hea or Cenegenics, who are well versed in the nuances of body compositi Be aware, however, that there are different types of DXA machines; t most recent versions specifically assess visceral body fat. Most sca are affordable and all produce very low dose radiation (similar to w you would receive from a cross-country flight from LA to NYC).

A useful quick measurement for obesity is waist circumferen Those patients with a waist circumference of >100 cm or 40 inc are likely obese and at risk for insulin resistance, and therefore DM Those with lower waist circumferences likely have not develop insulin resistance yet.

The important point is to move away from weight as a metric and focus more on body fat, particularly visceral fat stores.

Excess visceral fat is associated with high rates of heart disea DMII, and cancer. The critical factor is whether the fat has triggered inflammatory response in the body. This is an individual phenomen and can be influenced by many factors, such as genetics and exercis

However, it is important to note that the natural history of havi excess body fat is *that it will eventually cause inflammation*, so t those who carry excess fat but who are not currently inflamed sho still try to reduce their body fat.

Genetic Influence on Obesity

Little to none

Genetics can certainly influence metabolism to a small degree. For the most part, however, genetics is primarily important for cosmetic reasons, and is less of an influence on health.

People come in all different shapes and sizes. To the degree they affect cosmetics, genes are determining factors of leanness and body fat content.

From a health perspective, however, genetic variation in body fat is not significant, which makes sense for the long-term survival of the species. Except for uncommon pathologies such as Prader-Willi syndrome (a genetic deficiency of leptin) and other more rare syndromes, genetics is not a significant source of obesity for the average person. Genetics plays no role in the epidemic of obesity we are seeing now.

Simply put, genes are not the cause of obesity. Eating too much is. This is not to say that eating less is simple, it is obviously a monumental challenge. But, it is important not to get sidetracked. Genes cannot be blamed, except in that they compel us to eat when food is present.

Inflammation Overview

- *Inflammation is the cause of many chronic diseases*
- *Obesity contributes strongly to whole body inflammation*

Inflammation has been linked to many systemic disorders and is a critical factor in many (if not most) chronic diseases. Although allopathic medicine is excellent at treating acute surgical pathologies, it has well documented limitations in treating chronic illnesses. A large part of the limits of allopathic medicine relate to lack of effective preventions and interventions for addressing low but damaging levels of unresolved chronic inflammation.

Systemic inflammation is associated with other indicators of poor health: high cholesterol and waist circumference.

Inflammation is the source of arterial disease and is directly implicated in autoimmune disorders like multiple sclerosis.

The details of inflammation can be daunting to discuss, so we will limit our dialogue to those concepts that we believe are central to the understanding of age-related diseases.

The most useful way to think about inflammation is not in terms of good or bad, but rather in terms of balance and healing.

A certain degree of inflammation is required to heal, rebuild, and strengthen; very similar to the concept of *eustress*. Eustress, as opposed to *distress*, is a stress than strengthens. A simple example is a hard, but not crushing, workout at the gym. Another example can be the stress of academic study—the rigorous analyses that build and sharpen your ability to understand problems and find solutions. The body uses inflammation response to heal all kinds of insults, such as a cut to the skin surface. Other insults might come in the form of unhealthy foods we eat, which create oxidative stress and can potentially damage liver, endothelium, and nerve cells. The body uses inflammation as the "clean-up and repair team" at sites of insult or injury.

There are generally three phases of inflammation: The first is an acute (fast acting) vascular phase, followed by a more chronic cellular phase, and then a resolution phase.

The acute phase can be thought of as a cleanup phase. The cellular phase is a rebuilding phase, and the resolution phase is when the team leaves the scene, a pack-up phase. In many cases of chronic damaging inflammation, the cleanup team just never gets their act together to pack it in and leave the site. Sometimes this is because the site never gets rebuilt properly; we see this in many athletes who have chronic repetitive injuries that never quite heal (such as tennis elbow). Other times, the inflammatory response is overly active and the signals needed to tell the team to go home never get sent or received properly. In all cases, the inflammation is essentially unresolved.

Resolution of imbalanced chronic inflammation

The net balance of inflammation is sometimes reflected in laboratory tests your doctor might order. Other tests are more specific to a type of inflammation, like rheumatoid factor in some patients with rheumatoid arthritis. In general, we live under conditions that promote inflammation (stress, obesity, lack of exercise, poor sleep, and processed food products). Therefore, perhaps more than any other time in human history, we need to be even more vigilant about monitoring inflammation and promoting actions that reduce inflammation. The science of monitoring inflammation is still in its infancy, but we know a lot about how to reduce it.

Inflammation, Obesity, and Insulin Resistance

Obesity is directly related to inflammation—both cause and effect. Insulin resistance is central to the effect of obesity. Insulin resistance precedes DMII. As this chain of events evolves, if left unchecked, *metabolic syndrome* is likely to emerge. Metabolic syndrome is a substantial risk factor for increased heart disease related mortality because it describes an intermediary state of one or more clinical conditions that come before the formal diagnosis of DMII, which is strongly implicated in many cases of premature heart disease.

> ***Metabolic syndrome is comprised of obesity, a trend toward insulin resistance, hypertension, and bad cholesterol levels—all consequences of excess body fat.***

Leptin plays a major role in appetite regulation, as do incretins and insulin. Thus, inflammation and hormone insensitivity (insulin, leptin and incretins) play a major role in poorly controlled appetites.

Obesity creates inflammation because fat cells produce pro-inflammatory agents. We also observe infiltration into fat tissue by inflammatory cells such as macrophages and a disruption of lipid and sugar metabolism in obesity.

Fat Is a Pro-Inflammatory Endocrine Organ

- *Fat cells in healthy people secrete fewer inflammatory agents.*
- *Fat cells in obese people secrete more harmful inflammatory agents*

Like muscle, body fat is largely an endocrine organ; it is not just used for storing fats. Over 50 hormones, called adipocytokines, are described and categorized as either pro- or anti-inflammatory. Thus, we need to clarify the fact that fat is, in fact, an inflammatory gland, but not always secreting a net balance of harmful inflammatory agents. In fact, fat cells in a lean healthy person secrete more anti-inflammatory agents. In contrast, fat cells in an obese person secrete a net balance of harmful inflammatory agents.

The distribution or location of fat on your body often reflects a tendency toward heart disease. The amount of visceral fat you have around your middle strongly predicts your risk of heart disease. The total amount of body fat is also an important factor in determining if your fat cells secrete molecules that are harmful to your metabolism. Higher body fat leads to a different profile of the type of adipocytokines they secrete. Thus, fat cell type, distribution, and amount relative to lean body mass are important determinants of the net effect of body fat. Not all fat cells are the same. As you tax your fat cells to store more and more fat, they start to secrete more harmful inflammatory molecules.

In contrast, lean people secrete a disproportionate amount of anti-inflammatory agents from adipocytes. With a very low calorie diet, we know that more beneficial anti-inflammatory agents tend to be secreted by your fat cells, instead of harmful pro-inflammatory agents.

A month following a low-calorie diet has been shown to significantly reduce pro-inflammatory agents and increase anti-inflammatory agents—an impressive result in such a short period of time.

Inflammation directly and indirectly interferes with insulin action. As we now know, insulin resistance precedes DMII. We now turn our discussion to the topic of insulin and leptin resistance and how inflammation is tied to both.

Inflammation, obesity, insulin, & leptin resistance

Hormone insensitivity is commonly observed in obese patients, a trend worth tracking, because more studies will likely continue to show blunted responses of many hormones in obese or otherwise unhealthy people. When a patient is "insensitive" to a hormone, early on they will have high levels of that hormone circulating, in an attempt to compensate for less effective action. So, patients who develop DMII show elevated insulin, until later stages where insulin is not secreted because the pancreas is exhausted. We have recently discovered obese patients are also often leptin resistant, and we think this is directly related to inflammation in the hypothalamus.

Chronic inflammation of the hypothalamus is often thought to result in a new "set point" of weight.

There is a strong tendency for each of us to maintain our own weight. You might be able to identify your own set point by the relatively consistent weight you maintained before middle age. In obese patients, it is likely that the chronic inflammation of the hypothalamus in the brain results in a different set point. Once a new set point is established it becomes very difficult to reset it, which might partly explain why it is so difficult for most of us to sustain weight change after a short period of weight loss (7–8 months). Interestingly, even when we gain lean muscle, our bodies tend to stay the same weight, which means that body fat must go down. One of the strategies in our program is to increase lean tissue content (primarily bone and muscle), which usually results in body fat reduction, by virtue of the set point principle.

Muscle burns much more energy than fat does, as we will discuss in later sections. This is an added bonus to developing more lean tissue.

What can you do to reduce your body fat and risk of long-term disease?

- *To reduce body fat: Eat less*
- *To reduce inflammation: Eat better quality foods*

You now understand how obesity is the beginning of a cascade of problems that lead to premature heart disease (the biggest killer worldwide) and premature death. Inflammation and hormone resistance are consistently implicated in the molecular mechanisms along this course. But what can you do about it?

If you are overweight, drop the fork. Losing weight is most closely related to how much you eat, rather than exercise. Exercise has great benefits, discussed in the relevant chapter, but it usually results in more food intake to compensate for the increased energy expenditure.

For men, body fat of <20% is a target. We do not use BMI measurements. We try to get your visceral fat level to <20% because visceral fat is so closely linked with heart disease. We think it is reasonable to start with a target of 20% total body fat, then zero-in on visceral fat measurements. For women, who usually carry more body fat, we recommend a target of <25% body fat. Weight loss improves insulin resistance if it is put into practice early enough (before substantial resistance to insulin is established).

Again, we want to emphasize that it is the net balance of inflammation, not a particular measure of body fat or weight that is important.

Visceral body fat measurements are a good marker of the likelihood of future heart disease. Attempts should be made to keep it as low as possible.

Nutritionally, low-inflammation diets are optimal. In truth, there is nothing novel about a low inflammatory diet. It is a diet made up of whole foods. Studies have examined polyunsaturated fats (PUFAs) in detail. Nearly universally, results show PUFAs have anti-inflammatory features. In addition, omega-3 fatty acids (a type of PUFA) are likely at the core of the anti-inflammatory effects, whereas omega-6 fatty acids (also PUFAs) have more pro-inflammatory effects. They work synergistically, so do not try to eliminate all omega-6 fatty acids from your diet. Chances are, however, that your diet has plenty of omega-6 already in it. A 4:1 ratio of omega-6 to omega-3 is often recommended as ideal, if you can keep track of your fatty acids in such detail. Some experts recommend a 1:1 ratio. In any case, when you run into someone challenging PUFA's (omega-3 especially) healthfulness, take a hard look at the evidence they bring to the table. It is probably flawed.

Vitamin D's impact on inflammation is less certain, at least in the lab. Various studies do not support vitamin D improving insulin sensitivity and show no effect of supplemental vitamin D on inflammatory agents or insulin resistance. However, this is not to dismiss the importance of vitamin D. Vitamin D levels in healthy people tend to be much higher than in unhealthy people, and studies have shown that it is supportive of the immune system. It is also necessary for helping maintain strong bones. Besides, sunshine is good for the soul and probably has many positive effects we have yet to measure.

Statins have been used in copious amounts in an attempt to improve patients' cholesterol levels. However, there are important adverse effects to be aware of, one of which includes an increased risk of developing DMII.

We do not support the use of statin therapy as a primary prevention tool, but do recognize it might be helpful for high-risk patients for whom nutrition and exercise are not bringing about the progress a patient needs. Statins do have anti-inflammatory properties that can account for their positive impact on heart disease, rather than cholesterol profile changes.

Aspirin has often been used for primary prevention in aging patients to guard against heart disease risk. It has anti-inflammatory properties, and there is evidence to suggest it improves insulin sensitivity and cholesterol metabolism as well. However, the evidence is still mixed on its primary prevention benefits. Again, primary prevention is a term we use to describe something that is done before a problem exists. For example, a nutrition prescription to increase green leafy vegetable and wild fish consumption would be considered a primary prevention prescription.

Table 2.1

Anti-inflammatory and Pro-inflammatory Foods

Anti-inflammatory	Pro-inflammatory
Omega-3 fatty acids (wild fish)	Omega-6 fatty acids (fast food)
Spices (garlic, ginger, turmeric)	Refined and processed foods
Many nuts (walnuts, cashews, almonds)	Red meat and saturated fat
Green leafy vegetables	Grains

Macronutrients — Part III

Introduction

We now focus on how nutrition impacts conditions that precede heart disease. *Macronutrient* is a term used to describe 3 major energy sources found in food: carbohydrates, fats, and proteins. Carbohydrates are essentially sugar molecules. Proteins are composed of amino acids. There are about 20 amino acids in humans, about 10 of which are essential amino acids. We think you should consider fiber as the fourth macronutrient group, but a full discussion on the topic is beyond the scope of this version of the book.

Not all carbohydrates are the same; not all fats are the same; not all proteins are the same. Each subtype of macronutrient can have substantially different metabolic consequences. They act differently in the body. For example, fats are comprised of essential and nonessential fatty acids. Essential fatty acids are further comprised of PUFAs, some of which can be anti-inflammatory omega-3 fatty acids or pro-inflammatory omega-6 fatty acids.

> ***With a deeper understanding of how different carbohydrates, fats, and proteins signal metabolic function and appetite regulation, it becomes clear that sound nutrition is much more closely related to the modified truism of "we are what our body does with what we eat."***

So don't be fooled by food labels and media headlines about 'proteins" or "fats." Dig deeper to know which kinds of macronutrients hey are talking about. And stay away from sugar.

In food science, we often talk about the average energy obtained from "burning" a gram of fat or other macronutrient. These are estimates, not absolute numbers, of what kind of energy is released when such an amount is "burned." The table below gives you those numbers. They are not important once you get a handle on one simple fact. Fats are twice the calories as carbs and protein. It's that simple.

Table 3.1

The Established References for Energy Densities

Macronutrient	Energy Densities
Carbohydrates	4 kcal/g or 17 kJ/g
Fats	9 kcal/g or 39 kJ/g
Protein	4 kcal/g or 17 kJ/g

Adapted from Health and Welfare Canada

Carbohydrates

Reduce carbs and you will reduce insulin surges

The low-carb diet is the hottest macronutrient craze out there in the media and diet world, replacing the low-fat craze. The carb craze is here to stay, however, unlike the fat craze, which can be traced to a single misunderstood/misrepresented study by Ancel Keys. The low carb craze is based on science—thousands of articles ranging from molecular mechanisms to population data.

We know carbs are turned into fat, unless you are actively burning energy (for instance, if you are an athlete). So if you think you are avoiding becoming fat by eating carbs in place of fat or protein, you are unfortuntely mistaken.

Carbs are the only non-essential macronutrient. Fats and proteins are required for life; carbs are not. Much ongoing research is confirming what many have already discovered through athletics, bodybuilding, and weight loss efforts. The more we understand how body fat is actually an inflammatory endocrine organ, the more we realize excess carbs contribute most easily to body fat building. However, there is more to understand before we convince you the low-carb diet is not a fad.

As we have said, all carbs are not all the same. Some are worse than others, depending on how quickly (and how long) insulin levels are raised by the carb you eat. Apart from athletes in active training, we strongly recommend a low-carbohydrate food plan. In truth, it's not a "low-carb" diet; what we are saying is just "cut back on eating excessively highly processed carbs." One of the biggest complaints we hear about low-carb diets is that patients feel tired. At first, that might be true as your body adjusts its metabolism to accommodate the higher protein diet that compensates for the lower carbs. Very low-carb diets (<20 g) are often too low to tolerate for long.

You don't need 200 g a day of carbs to feel good, to be active, and to have zip in the boardroom. On the contrary, eating that many carbs will drain you of energy, increase inflammation, and not satisfy your appetite.

Low carb is define as an intake of absolutely less than 150 grams per day. However, we start patients on a 20-50 grams of carbohydrates per day diet for a month, and then add back healthy carbs (such as leafy veggies) to provide for training or other activity-related needs. Most people are very comfortable on 100 g/day of carbs, most of which are derived from vegetables.

We never recommend more than 150 grams of carbs per day because carbs are about 4 kcal of energy per gram consumed—so that 150 g still amounts to 600 kcal. If the average non-athlete diet is 2000 kcal, then a 150 g carbohydrate diet would still consist of about 30% carbs. A very low-carb diet is 20 g/day or about 4% of total energy. Nobody is particularly happy on a diet below 20 g/day, so we never even suggest it. We want changes to be sustainable, tolerable, and add value to the quality of life of people we care for, not detract from it. A reasonable diet is about 100 g of carbs/day and is very sustainable by a mildly health-conscientious person.

What exactly is a carb?

Sugar. In the end, all carbs become sugar (glucose) in your bloodstream

Glucose, fructose, and galactose (all sugar) are the simplest forms of carbohydrates. The longer the chain of glucose the carb is made of, then the more complex the carb. But complexity doesn't mean it is healthy. It might mean it is slightly less unhealthy, but don't drink the Kool-Aid that a "complex carb" is good for you.

All carbs are eventually converted into sugar by the body. Sugar is used as the primary source of energy in most tissue cells throughout the body, including the muscle and brain. Your body only has around 40 kcals of sugar in the bloodstream at any given time (the equivalent of around three teaspoons of table sugar), and the body will try to defend going above this level rigorously. It does so primarily by turning sugar into fat. Given the rather limited tolerance your body has for sugar in the bloodstream, it is quite easy to exceed this level.

The liver is an integral component to metabolizing simple sugars by storing them as glycogen (super long chains of stored sugar) before then storing them as fatty acids in fat cells.

The pancreas is instrumental in helping all tissues take up glucose into their cells by secreting insulin, which "pushes sugar into cells." When energy deficiencies exist, they are replenished with food intake. When food intake occurs despite the fact you don't have an energy deficiency, then fat cells are used to store that energy.

Why fewer carbs?

Burn fewer carbs, burn more fat

From a health perspective, carbohydrates have several direct negative results. Insulin surges are created from almost all carbohydrates—even "complex" carbohydrates such as whole-wheat bread, and whole-grain corn chips. Do not be fooled by packaging and marketing efforts. Carbohydrates are quickly converted into fatty acids that are then stored in fat cells. So, unless you have just fasted or exercised to a point where your muscle cells are depleted of stored carbohydrates (called glycogen), then the carb you eat is going to be stored as a fat cell. We will tell you more about why body fat (beyond 20% for men and 25% for women) is unhealthy. In the meantime, the insulin surge created from the carbohydrate contributes to the development of DMII. The more insulin surges you have, the more likely you are to develop DMII. Additionally, carbohydrates are not appetite-satisfying. Protein is the most effective hunger stopping macronutrient. Fats are also satiating, but are the easiest macronutrient to be added to a fat cell as a TG. Once TGs are stored, it takes stress to get them released. You are better off eating healthy proteins or fats (such as omega-3 fatty acids) than a bunch of carbs.

The only carbohydrates that we recommend are those from vegetables, avoiding white vegetables (such as potatoes), peas (a legume, not a vegetable), and soybeans (because of the overabundance of soy in processed food).

Green leafy vegetables have a powerful combination of healthy fiber and great nutrient value, with very few carbs. Eat them up—spinach and kale and all of their amazing varieties. These green leafy vegetables are packed full of so many nutrients we know are great for you and many other nutrients we might not even know about yet. As an added bonus—of the few carbs that come out of kale, a good portion of them are used just to digest the green leafy power-packed vegetable.

Fruits are certainly better than chips (any kind of chip, including organic blue corn, whole grain, sesame seed-laden chips). We advocate 2 to 3 servings of fruit per day in most cases. However, fruits will still produce considerably higher insulin surges than healthy vegetables. The sugar in fruit is almost always fructose, which is a relatively simple sugar compared with the very complex carbohydrates found in vegetables. Thus, the insulin surges are higher, with all of the consequences of an insulin surge. Given a choice between a fruit and a vegetable, a vegetable is usually healthier. But, given the choice of a fruit or packaged snacks, the fruit is clearly a better choice.

We suggest to patients to avoid grains entirely, including quinoa and other "healthier" options. If you do indulge, do so knowing that regardless of the labeling, the "whole" grain you are eating is almost certainly not whole. The vast majority of the products called whole grain are legally allowed to claim the term because they put back the endosperm, bran, and germ after it had been processed out. Most manufacturers will start with a whole grain product that requires processing. After the processing, to make a non-whole grain product whole grain again, the manufacturer adds back the separated ingredients; a procedure perfectly sanctioned by the FDA.

How are carbs, blood sugar levels, and insulin related?

The glycemic load is the effect sugar you eat has on insulin surges

When carbohydrates are eaten, they are broken down in the gut (small intestine) to simple sugars—usually glucose. The sugar enters the bloodstream from the gut. The body wants blood sugar levels to be low because, among other reasons, circulating glucose damages the lining of small blood vessels and interferes with things such as hemoglobin, the molecule that carries oxygen. So, in order to keep blood sugar low, as soon as glucose enters the bloodstream, it is "pushed" into cells like the muscle and liver, to rebuild lost stores of glycogen. Insulin is the hormone that pushes glucose into those cells. If there is plenty of stored sugar present in the cell already, oxidative cell damage can occur when insulin tries to push too much glucose into the cell. Oxidative cell damage places that cell's DNA at risk for mutations and cancer development. Ultimately, the circulating blood sugar that cannot fit into muscle or other cells will be stored in fat cells as TGs. TGs then go on to change your cholesterol levels, but that is another story. The more overcrowded fat cells become, the more they secrete pro-inflammatory (unhealthy) molecules, as we discussed in the section on obesity. Fat cells become overstuffed with TGs; these essentially become an endocrine gland that secretes pro-inflammatory molecules. Therefore, minimizing insulin surges is paramount to your health.

The size of the sugar molecule *partly* influences the speed of digestion and blood sugar/insulin elevation, but not entirely. Other factors that influence the speed of digestion include the presence of other nutrients or fiber consumed, the preparation method, and individual genetic differences in metabolizing the nutrients.

Understanding how what you eat influences blood sugar and then insulin elevation (the insulinogenic effect) is essential in reframing how you see the healthfulness of your food. Eating a carbohydrate causes three processes to occur:

- An ingested carbohydrate will become glucose
- Blood glucose will become elevated
- To reduce blood glucose, insulin levels will rise

One thing to keep in mind, however, as you continue to try to push sugar into your cells, is that your cells "push back" and become resistant to insulin. Insulin resistance is your cells' way of trying to minimize damage caused by trying to store too much sugar. Fat cells are for storing energy. But when they get overstuffed, they start secreting pro-inflammatory agents.

How do we measure sugar-induced insulin surges in the food you eat?

There are three ways we use to help describe the insulin-elevating effects of foods:

Glycemic index
Correlates well with insulin response from theoretical amounts of sugar in your food.

Glycemic load
Correlates well with insulin response from realistic amounts of sugar in your food.

Food insulin index (FII)
Not yet a fully developed system, but most directly correlates with insulin response to sugar in your food.

Understanding GL is probably the most useful concept to develop. We do not advocate for routine counting of the GI or GL of your food, though initially you will want to become familiar with what foods are high- or low-GL. Then you will have a foundation for an understanding of what you eat and how it affects your insulin response, which is the first step in making better food choices—recognizing the true nutritional value of what is sold to you and what you eat.

Glycemic index

Useful in developing the concept of linking carbs to insulin surges

The GI of a food product measures how fast your blood sugar levels rise after eating 50 g of a carbohydrate source. White bread has the same GI as pure sugar, and therefore is often used as a reference. Both white bread and sugar are assigned a GI of 100. GI values from other foods are referenced against the GI of white bread or sugar, and are less than 100. Databases exist to estimate the GI of any single food item, including http://www.glycemicindex.com. You might be surprised at what food items have high glycemic indices.

The drawback of GI values is that they do not account for a typical serving amount. For example, the GI of watermelon is 72, if you eat 50 g of it. Most people do not eat 50 g of watermelon in one sitting (about 5 cups). So realistically, your body will probably experience a much lower elevation of glucose when you eat a serving of watermelon. GI is still useful, conceptually, because it helps us understand GL.

Glycemic load

The most useful concept of all three, because it considers fiber and the typical amount of food eaten

The GL incorporates the amount of a typical serving of a given food product when considering the expected effect on blood glucose levels. Therefore, it more accurately reflects daily eating patterns. GL is most commonly calculated from the GI.

GL= (GI* ingested amount of carbs in g)/100

Other hormones besides insulin respond to elevated blood sugar

Incretins are higher with high blood sugar

High GL also leads to high levels of incretins, hormones that lower blood sugar by stimulating further insulin secretion, and cause fat to be stored. Thus, high GL foods are something you want to avoid.

Table 3.2

Glycemic Load Ranges

GL	Range
Low	<10
Medium	10–20
High	≥20

**Adapted from Livesey et al.*

Food insulin index

Too complex to use, but highlights the challenge of predicting insulin surges

The FII is a score of insulin levels based on a standard 240 kcal (a small meal) intake of a specific food. The score is compared to the insulin response shown when eating white bread (FII=100).

One of the most important things we have learned by studying FII, however, is that baked sweets and meats (beef and processed meats like hot dogs, bacon, and lunch meats) have high insulin indices. We also have confirmed what we thought we knew, which is breakfast cereals (like Cheerios) and oatmeal still have very high insulin responses. As expected, vegetables and real nuts produce negligible insulin scores.

So why does GI/GL matter?

Many studies show lower GI/GL food plans result in better health by reducing the following chronic diseases:

- Obesity
- Insulin resistance
- Type 2 diabetes
- Heart disease

How does eating low GI/GL food result in better health?

By reducing carbohydrates you reduce blood sugar levels, which does the following:

- Reduces insulin surges
- Reduces free radical production that can lead to cancer
- Increases nitric oxide production in blood vessels, promoting better blood flow
- Reduces protein glycation, which is associated with many age-related chronic diseases
- Reduces blood vessel damage
- Reduces oxidative stress that damages cells

Indirect benefits of a low GI/GL diet (by default you eat more fat, protein, and fiber):

- Protein and healthy fats make you feel more satisfied after a meal, promoting longer periods between meals
- Protein especially promotes heat production, which results in a higher overall metabolism (baseline level of energy use is higher)
- Fat is used as fuel
- Higher fiber in the diet aids digestion

- Less inflammation
- Higher HDL (generally considered a good fat)
- Harmful TG levels are lower

Summary of GI/GL

Many experimental, well-designed studies have repeatedly demonstrated that reduced GL food intake improves body fat loss, reduces insulin sensitivity, promotes a more favorable cholesterol profile, and reduces heart disease risk factors. Lower carbohydrates are good for you.

Mechanisms for how a lower GL diet helps you include that you feel fuller longer after a meal, you develop a higher metabolic rate, and have lower elevations of blood sugar and insulin surges after eating.

> ***Perhaps one of the most powerful benefits of reducing GL, and therefore insulin surges, is that your body starts burning fat for fuel—so you become a fat burner instead of a fat builder.***

However, you do not have to go to extremes to reach a lower GL diet. We suggest everyone target a carbohydrate intake of not more than 150 g per day. It is not unreasonable, unless you are an athlete in training. But once you target a quantifiable level, start shifting the sources of carbohydrates from bread and snack products to fruits and better yet, vegetables. We advocate a low and *slow* carbohydrate food plan, primarily comprised of fibrous vegetables; it will nearly eliminate your risk of DMII. For those of you who might be in the first stages of DMII, a low GL might save you from progressing or even reverse your metabolic state to a nondiabetic condition. You can cure yourself by eating lower GL foods.

We apply the concept of GI/GL in the first phase of treatment, with the same principles to be later applied by you to your independent decision making regarding food intake. We encourage you to *not to eat anything made of grains or white vegetables*. But do not get too caught up in exact measurements of GI/GL. A general reduction in high-GI foods is what you are aiming for.

Practically applied, we are simply trying to help you gather tools that can be used to create improvements in metabolism, which tends to be linked to reduced body fat. GI, GL, intermittent fasting, meal frequency, reduction of alcohol intake, meal replacement products, macronutrient combinations, and exercise are all simply tools that can be applied singularly or in combination to further goals. The usefulness of these tools is reflected in your preferences and ability to achieve a reasonable compliance. ***Compliance is king.***

Insulin: A Carbohydrate-Responsive Hormone

Insulin is the common link between carbohydrates and fat metabolism

Insulin surges build body fat

Insulin builds fat. Ultimately, it takes excess carbohydrates that won't fit into your muscle or liver and stores them as TGs in your fat cells. You can think of insulin pushing sugar for energy into cells, but it also redirects excess sugar into those fat cells.

Insulin also makes fat cells "greedy"—so to speak. In an environment of high insulin, fat cells are less willing to release their stored fatty acids in the form of TGs, so insulin impedes your fat being used as fuel. In fact, when insulin levels are kept low, you are in the fat burning zone. The lower your insulin levels stay, the exponentially greater you burn fat. Figure 3.1 illustrates that concept. Thus, at low insulin levels, releasing and burning fat becomes the preferred method of energy use.

You can see why it's hard to burn fat when insulin levels keep surging. Have you ever had a friend tell you he has cut back on eating? He will swear he is eating less, but he just can't seem to drop the weight, right? Well, he might still be eating too many carbs. Carbs directly inhibit fat burning because they cause insulin surges. So, he can't drop the weight (meaning body fat) because instead of eating lean animal protein sources like chicken and fish, he's still eating burgers and big buns. Instead of eating chips, maybe he switched to low-fat cookies. Low-fat is not going to reduce the carbs. Low-fat means high sugar.

The way to burn fat is to reduce insulin levels. Keep the insulin surges to a minimum and the fat will burn. Figure 3.1 shows why.

Figure 3.1

Lower Your Insulin—*Become a Fat Burner* Rather Than a Fat Builder

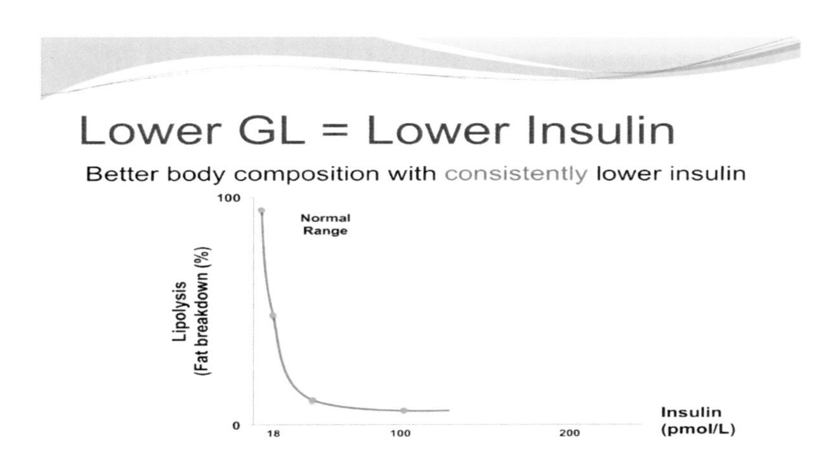

So what else does insulin do besides promote body fat accumulation?

How do insulin surges make you a fat builder instead of a fat burner?

- Insulin directly promotes fat production (lipogenesis)
- Insulin stops breakdown (lipolysis)
- Insulin stops fat from being used as fuel (β oxidation)

Your circulating cholesterol levels are negatively affected by insulin surges

Insulin surges create more TGs, as we discussed above. Both TGs and cholesterol circulate in the bloodstream by hanging onto a lipoprotein molecule. The lipoprotein is what we measure when we measure he "bad" low-density lipoprotein (LDL), the "good" high-density ipoprotein (HDL), and subsets of these molecules. Lipoproteins are ike a minibus and cholesterol and TGs are like the passengers. TGs ake up much more room on the bus than cholesterol. They also displace the cholesterol, which means more lipoproteins (the minibus) must be made to carry the unseated cholesterol. Both TGs and cholesterol need the bus. So when do elevated TGs start competing for bus seats?

TG levels go up with carbohydrate intake. Thus, circulating lipoprotein levels go up with carbohydrate intake. We used to think eating saturated fat increased the cholesterol in your bloodstream. We were wrong. This myth is discussed later. In fact, the more *carbs* you eat, the worse your cholesterol profile is. A worse cholesterol profile means a higher cholesterol level, as well as a less healthy cholesterol mix.

It's true that the worse your cholesterol levels, the more *likely* you are to have a heart attack. However, you should keep in mind an interesting point about heart attacks: Most people who have heart attacks have "normal" cholesterol levels. We explain why shortly.

Summary: Insulin

You now understand how insulin surges lead to fat building. Over time, to protect themselves, your cells will become insensitive to insulin. Once insensitivity begins, DMII is right around the corner for many. Moreover, reducing insulin and incretin surges promotes many good things. In short, lower GL reduces insulin-related inflammation and pancreatic β-cell stress, and promotes fatty acid fuel use, instead of storage. Lower insulin surges means you are a Fat Burner, instead of a Fat Builder. Daily lower insulin response is ideal for healthy living.

DMII risk and excess carbohydrates

The more carbohydrates you eat, the more likely you are to develop DMII

The state of DMII is entirely preventable for the vast majority of people who have it. For some, it can be reversed. Essentially, DMII is a state of insensitivity to hormones such as insulin and incretins. It stops sugar from being removed from the bloodstream. Sugar circulating in the blood vessels damages them, which is why DMII is essentially a vascular disease.

The risk of DMII increases with high-sugar (GL) food plans. Specifically, those who eat high-GL diets have a 250% increased risk of developing DMII. Those who have a moderate-GL food plan have a 26% risk of developing DMII.

> ***GL is a reflection of the quality of the carbohydrate, and vegetables (not potatoes) have a negligible GL. Fruits are nearly negligible in GL.***

Very low GI/GL diets (<20 g/day) are associated with lower markers of DMII and more weight loss. Although it is not reasonable to sustain this type of food plan, it does provide further support that reduced GL food plans promote health.

Heart disease risk increases with carbohydrates

The risk of heart disease is increased with high-GL diets. People who eat high-GL diets have twice the risk of developing heart disease.

Summary: Carbohydrates

Our new patients with weight loss goals are initially started on a very low carbohydrate diet during their induction phase. Motivation is high when they start a new program. The results of the diet are usually consistent, and the duration is tolerable for most (30 days).

Maintaining such a diet is impractical, however, and is of dubious long term benefit. Our goal, over time, is to add back complex healthy (low-GL) carbohydrate sources while causing few, if any, insulin surges. With increased body awareness, you can establish your individual ideal carb intake level, allowing you to manage your food intake for your desired body composition.

The degree of carbohydrate restriction you require is based on you and your strengths or weaknesses in three primary domains: glycemic control, weight management, and inflammation.

The first domain is glycemic control. In people with diabetes and pre-diabetes or anyone with insulin insensitivity issues, it is simply absurd to continue to challenge your system with any carbohydrate that provokes an insulin response. This, from a practical standpoint, means all carbohydrates would come from vegetables and perhaps one or two servings of fibrous fruits.

The second domain is weight management. Anyone with fat loss goals will want to restrict energy-dense carbohydrates, simply to reduce caloric intake. You have to eat less to lose body fat. Weight comes off quicker when the limited calories you do consume come from low-GL foods. In part, this is because you create a low insulin environment that allows fat to be the body's preferred fuel source.

The third domain relates to inflammation. Here, grains (particularly wheat) and dairy are the more common offenders. Joint pain, rhinitis, eczema, dry skin, fatigue, GERD, and other gastrointestinal disturbances are very commonly due to food sensitivities. Although not life threatening, they can degrade your quality of life significantly.

Athletic populations need more carbohydrates in the diet, and even those who do not have particular weaknesses in these domains should strive to make vegetables their first source of carbohydrates, followed by fibrous fruit.

As we will see later, each person has an individual response to altering the macronutrient mix. It is the nature of the individual response that requires individual attention from knowledgeable care providers, nutritionists, and exercise experts, to optimize your health, and learn about how your body works.

Fats

Over the past 5–8 years, it has become glaringly obvious that fat is not the culprit in causing heart attacks or heart disease. Yes, elevated lipoprotein levels are present in many patients with heart disease, but not all. Furthermore, we just explained how elevated blood sugar levels lead to elevated TG levels, which leads to more circulating lipoproteins, thus explaining the elevated LDL levels we see in patients at risk of heart disease.

The terminology of fats is often confusing and misused, even among care providers. We will highlight the most important categories of fats as they relate to your health.

In general, when we discuss fats, we are talking about fatty acids. They can be classified as saturated or unsaturated.

Saturated vs. unsaturated fat

MYTH of Saturated Fats

Myth: ***Saturated fatty acids are the major culprit in heart disease.***

Fact: ***Carbohydrates are the culprit in heart disease.***

Many myths in medicine start with "landmark" studies that propose theories from either misrepresented or misinterpreted data. Incorrect conclusions are drawn that can take years, if not decades, to reverse—incurring enormous costs to produce the necessary high-powered studies to reverse the current theory.

Heart disease is indisputably the largest contributor to death in the both the US and globally. More people die from heart disease than any other cause. Cancers, as a diverse group, are a close second.

Decades ago, saturated fat was presented as the reason why people had heart attacks and developed heart disease. Cholesterol (LDL-C and HDL-C) levels were was presented as markers that determined how high your risk was.

Ancel Keys is credited for presenting the first correlative data that would wrongly convince the scientific community that saturated fats are potentially causative of heart disease. His initial paper on the positive correlation of saturated fat intake and cardiovascular mortality selectively used data from 7 countries, when data was available for 22. When all 22 countries were included in the data, the significance of the findings was reduced (but not eliminated). It is important to understand that studies like these, on large populations of people, show a relationship (correlation).

Correlation does mean something caused it, though many times an author will want to imply that with headlines. The correlation between heart attacks and saturated fat means we find people who have heart attacks (and develop heart disease) also eat a lot saturated fat. Just because we find a common thread of increased saturated fat intake with heart disease, it does not mean the saturated fats cause heart disease. In fact, it doesn't.

However, the correlation made intuitive sense, right? Eat fat, get fat in the bloodstream, and get heart disease. It isn't so simple, for two big reasons. The first is that eating lots of fat does not necessarily result in higher fat in the bloodstream. The second is that **heart disease starts with blood vessel damage caused by inflammation.** Heart disease is not caused by fat clogging pipes at the beginning. **Clogged pipes are the end result of damaged blood vessels being exposed to circulating fat.**

Let's discuss how cholesterol (a type of fat) circulates in the bloodstream. Circulating particles call lipoproteins are made in the liver to carry cholesterol. The lipoproteins are the LDL and HDL blood tests your doctor orders to help assess your risk of heart disease. Think of lipoproteins as the minibuses that carry cholesterol. Lipoproteins are made by the liver. You might think that eating dietary fat, such as cheese, causes more cholesterol (riding on the lipoproteins) to be made.

It turns out, cholesterol production increases with excess carbohydrate intake; not excess fat intake.

Why is that? It is because two different molecules actually ride on the lipoprotein bus—cholesterol and TGs. Because TGs are elevated with excess carbohydrate intake and insulin surges, excess carbs mean more lipoproteins to accommodate the higher TG levels (that get shuttled into fat cells for a rainy day). Lipoproteins, like LDL and HDL (and variations) are used to tell us how high your risk is for a heart attack. So carbohydrate intake, not fat, determines your heart attack risk.

We are not saying saturated fats are healthy. They are not healthy in excess of 7% of your diet. But they do not cause heart disease. Carbohydrates and bad lifestyle choices do (such as smoking and excessive alcohol consumption). It is probably the other unhealthy behaviors that we see in the people who also eat a lot of saturated fat in

Western cultures that contributes to premature heart attacks. The good news is that because most (but not all) saturated fats come from dairy and animal meat, they are easy to minimize. But make no mistake, they do not cause heart disease. Carbohydrates do. In fact, we also now know there is no correlation of dietary saturated fat intake and saturated fat in the bloodstream. It is well established in studies decades after we said the opposite.

Anecdotally, many cultures have a high percentage of saturated fats in their diets, including native Alaskans (75% of diet), the Maasai tribe in Africa (66% of diet), natives of Tokelau in the Pacific (60% of diet), and human breast milk, which consists of 54% saturated fat. The high saturated fat diets listed above, coupled with *un*saturated fat components and protein, implies approximately a 10%–30% carbohydrate diet—low to very low.

Later, we will more fully discuss the myth that has you thinking that heart disease is caused by vessel blockage, like a clogged pipe. It is not.

Myth: ***High cholesterol alone causes heart attacks***

Fact: ***Inflammation-damaged blood vessels and cholesterol cause heart attacks***

Cholesterol with endothelial damage creates blood vessel plaque, but cholesterol without endothelial damage does not. This helps to explain why most people who have a heart attack actually have normal cholesterol levels. In those people, the endothelial damage was substantial enough that even normal levels of cholesterol placed them at risk. It also helps to explain why some people with high levels of cholesterol do not experience a cardiac event—because they do not have substantial endothelial damage.

> ***Cholesterol does not cause plaque formation in someone with healthy blood vessels (healthy endothelium).***

Most endothelium is unhealthy because of inflammation. Therefore, higher cholesterol increases your risk of cardiac events because higher cholesterol increases your probability of having inflamed/damaged endothelium. Nutrition and exercise can both dramatically improve unhealthy endothelium and therefore reduce cardiac events. Yes, using medicine to lower cholesterol will reduce the probability of plaque simply because of a lower probability of interacting with damaged endothelium. However, the way to attack heart disease is from both sides, reducing cholesterol and improving endothelial health. Nutrition and Exercise create an effective double-pronged approach.

Essential fatty acids

Unsaturated fats: MUFAS and PUFAS

Unsaturated fats include essential and nonessential fats. For now we are going to focus on 2 unsaturated essential fatty acids (EFA).

If an unsaturated fat has one double bond in its molecule, it is called a MUFA- monounsaturated fatty acid (like in olive oil). MUFAs are not essential fatty acids, but they are often healthy.

If they are unsaturated fats and have 2 or more double bonds in their molecules, they are called PUFAs—polyunsaturated fatty acids. The two EFAs we will discuss are PUFAs.

Essential fats are specific types of unsaturated fats that need to be eaten because we cannot make them—that is why we call them essential. ALA and LA are essential. You can remember these two fats because ALA sort of sounds like alpha. LA sort of sounds like lay, or LEIC.

ALA is **alpha**-linolenic acid
LA is lino**LEIC** acid.

For reasons we get into later, one might be considered "good," the other "bad." In truth, the bad one is just misunderstood, as is often the case. Both are good for us, but one is an omega-3 fatty acid (like what you find in salmon and other fish oil). The other is an omega-6 fatty acid (like what you find more commonly in packaged food products or less healthy foods (grains, cereals, safflower oil, corn oil, mayo, soy). Check out the packages of food at the grocery store. These ingredients are rampant. The way we first remembered which was which is that alpha is at the top—and omega-3 fatty acids are certainly at the top of nutrients to put into your body. They rock. LA is lame, just another omega-6 fatty acid.

ALA omega-3 because it is Alpha
LA omega-6 because it is **Lame**

The thing is that we eat tons of omega-6 fatty acids already in our diet. There is no shortage. In fact, there is an excess of omega-6 fatty acid in most diets. We know that Paleolithic diets were composed of about an equal amount of omega-6 and omega-3 fatty acids. There is evidence to suggest an optimal ratio of omega-6 to omega-3 fatty acids can range from 3:2 to as high as 4:1. Today, many diets are 15:1 (omega-6:omega-3 fatty acids). Why is this not healthy? Although some omega-6 fatty acids are required to help omega-3 fatty acids act as anti-inflammatory agents, the general tendency is for omega-6 fatty acids is to be pro-inflammatory. Thus, when the balance is tipped toward omega-6 fatty acids, we are tipping the balance of inflammation to a more inflammatory state (pro-inflammatory).

The importance of balancing PUFAs (the omega 6:3 ratio)

PUFAs, like all macronutrients, cannot be viewed as a broad homogeneous group, but need to be approached individually. When a study says more PUFAs are not healthy for you, it might be correct. That is, increasing PUFAs as a group, without regard to how much omega-3 or omega-6 fatty acid is present, is nearly meaningless. PUFAs, as a group, include pro- and anti-inflammatory fats. If you increase a pro-inflammatory fat, like linoleic acid, it is no surprise that there are worse outcomes.

Omega-3 fatty acids, a very healthy form of a PUFA, are well established as anti-inflammatory. Omega-6 fatty acids are well established as pro-inflammatory. Therefore, not all PUFAs are the same.

The omega-6 to -3 ratio is often discussed because it seems to be important to balance intake of some omega-6 fats with lots of omega 3-fats. The ideal ratio that has been put forward is an omega 6:omega 3 ratio of $\leq$4:1.

Wild-caught salmon is well documented to contain lots more omega-3 fats than farm-raised salmon (which contain far more omega-6 fats).

Research indicates the diets of Paleolithic humans contained a 1:1 omega ratio. In fact, the Paleolithic human diet was dominated by omega-3 fatty acids in virtually all foods—meat, wild plants, eggs, fish, nuts, and berries. US diets consist of an approximately 15:1 omega ratio, instead of the 1:1 ratio Paleolithic humans ingested. The genetic difference between Paleolithic humans and modern humans is estimated at 0.005% difference—not likely enough difference to warrant such a dramatic change in nutritional needs.

Sources of omega-3 fatty acids include grass-fed beef and milk/butter products, wild or free-range animals, wild-caught coldwater fish (salmon, mackerel), and tuna (Albacore is best; avoid tuna canned in oil).

Sources of omega-6 fatty acids include corn oil, soy oil, canola oil, safflower oil, sunflower oil, and farm-raised animals (chickens, salmon, and tilapia—most of which is "made in China").

Until 50 years ago, DMII was exceedingly rare in Greenland. Greenland natives' diets are high in seafood and therefore high in omega-3 fatty acids. Such a diet is naturally associated with low rates of heart disease, diabetes mellitus I, multiple sclerosis, and asthma. Further study of omega-3 fatty acids has shown significant benefits in other diseases related to inflammation including inflammatory bowel disease, rheumatoid arthritis, psoriasis, and specific malignancies.

Tips to improve the omega ratio

- Eat more wild coldwater fish.
- Supplement with organic whole food sources, such as salmon.
- Use macadamia nut oil for cooking instead of olive oil.
- Reserve olive oil for room temperature use or cold dishes.

Nonessential FA

The evidence against trans fatty acids

This isn't even controversial. Don't eat processed foods that use them.

Food processing methods that create trans fats attempt to attain solid fat properties from liquid fat through partially hydrogenating it. The result is a type of trans fatty acid that has been unequivocally linked to causing a higher heart disease risk cholesterol profile—elevating LDL and lowering HDL. Additionally, trans fatty acids interfere with insulin receptors, promoting an insulin resistant state—DMII.

> ***Studies have convinced even the stoic FDA that trans fats are unhealthy and contribute substantially to heart disease.***

Sources of trans fats include partially hydrogenated vegetable oil (to make it more solid at room temperature), margarine, vegetable shortening, processed meats, fast foods, and manufactured and processed food products. The very small amount of trans fats that occur in nature are not necessarily the same as those created by food processing.

Myth: Zero trans fats on the label means that no trans fats are present

Fact: Zero trans fats per serving means you still might get a small amount of trans fats

The FDA allows the manufacturer to label a product "0 trans fats per serving" if the serving size contains less than 0.5 g of trans fats. The simple solution for the unscrupulous manufacturer is to create as many serving sizes as necessary to reduce the amount of trans fats to below 0.5 g, thus allowing them to label the package with 0 trans fats.

***Myth:* Oil heated to the smoking point contains lots more trans fats**

***Fact:* Oil heated to smoking tastes bad and is less healthy, but has only a non-significant, marginal increase in trans configured fats.**

The smoking point is the temperature at which oil burns or smokes. The smoking points referenced are generally created under optimal conditions; with increased exposure of the oil to light, and after the oil container has been opened, the smoking point will be lower. Antioxidants are damaged at the smoking point, thus an important component of nutritional value is lost. However, the amount of trans fats that can occur at the smoking point are negligible.

As a rule, olive oil should be used for cold foods, or placed upon warmed foods after cooking. Cooking with olive oil, especially lower-quality olive oils, can result in lost nutritional value.

Interesterified fatty acids (unsaturated): The new 'trans' fats?

Avoid products with interesterified fats for now

Interesterified fatty acids have essentially taken over the role in processed foods that trans fatty acids used to play. They are created from combining stearic acid (a saturated fat) with vegetable oils containing unsaturated fats. *Interesterified fats have also been shown to increase LDL, lower HDL, and increase blood glucose levels by 20%.* Although only small controlled trials have been performed to date, the evidence is compelling enough to warrant consumer avoidance.

A healthier alternative to both trans fatty acids and interesterified fatty acids, both of which are manufactured, is to use highly saturated, naturally occurring vegetable oils or saturated fats from animal products.

Either is healthier than the manufactured variations. Variations of palm oil (45% oleic or a high oleic variation at 55%) from the fruit of the palm plant are healthy alternatives because they contain antioxidants and vitamin E. Palm kernel and fractionated palm oil are to be avoided.

Selected topics of fat metabolism

Everyone has subtle variations in how they process food.

Some patients with different gene variants need lower dietary fat intake

One of the important concepts we have learned through clinical experience is that each person has subtle differences that accelerate or impede progress, in all domains (such as nutrition, exercise, and hormone optimizing). Current research is unveiling genetic influences that help to explain some of the variables that eluded us in years past. One such example relates to the APOε gene and the variable response we sometimes see to the statins used to lower "bad fat" levels in your bloodstream (recall the example of the bus).

> ***There is considerable controversy around statins, especially whether they should be used by everyone at a certain age, to prevent heart disease (primary prevention).***

We address this issue later in the book. For now, what is important to understand is that some people respond better to low-fat diets and statins than others. We now know part of the reason for the variable response has to do with the APOε gene.

The normal APOε gene is referred to as the APOε3. The one that has been strongly linked to Alzheimer's dementia (AD) is the APOε4. There is also an APOε2 gene. We have learned that people who have the APOε2 gene respond well to statins, but low-fat diets increase dense harmful small particle lipoproteins (lots of TGs riding on them make them denser). Such patients are recommended to consume a 35% fat diet. These patients also tend to respond to alcohol intake with high HDL and lower LDL.

Patients' specific genetic variations also play a role in who will respond more vigorously to LDL-lowering efforts. Lowering dietary saturated fats will have little effect on lowering LDL in women, patients who are obese, who have DMII, or who carry the common APOε3 allele.

Lowering dietary saturated fats will have an increased response to lowering LDL in patients with the APOε4 allele who are predisposed to a higher LDL level. Interestingly, the APOε4 allele is a common link between increased risk of dementia and increased risk of heart disease.

Summary: Fats

Fats are perhaps the most complex macronutrient. They directly influence the balance of inflammation in the body through well-established but complex pathways, and can be directly incorporated into cell membranes, thus providing a concrete example of the truism, "You are what your body does with what you eat (and what it ate or was fed)."

Unsaturated fats include nonessential fatty acids and essential fatty acids (EFA). Nonessential fatty acids include trans and interesterified fatty acids. The former is proven unhealthy and the latter has small clinical trials that suggest it is unhealthy as well. Both are created by the food industry to reduce costs (lowering nutrient value) and improve shelf appeal. Essential fatty acids (especially omega-3 fatty acids such as ALA) should be maximized in our diets, given far too much omega-6 is eaten daily. Data suggests an optimal diet would have a 1:1 ratio of omega-6:omega-3, but not greater than 4:1. Like essential amino acids, discussed in the next section, essential fatty acids must be eaten; the body cannot make them.

The quality of the food source largely depends on the material it was fed. Free-range animals are consistently healthier and often have demonstrably higher-quality fat content compared with farm-raised animals.

Omega-3 fatty acids are the defusing macronutrient. It is a strongly preferred fat source that we emphasize to patients to avoid providing the "fuse" of carbohydrates which tend to light the fat bomb. We emphasize controlling fat intake to the degree one needs to control energy intake (calorie density).

When evaluating fat intake, one must also specify the amount and type of carbohydrate and protein in the diet; not just how much fat or even how much saturated fat.

A low-carbohydrate approach, emphasizing vegetables and to a lesser extent fibrous fruits as the primary sources will allow a more simplified approach to fat intake.

The primary approach to fat intake is to emphasize whole food sources of omega-3 fats, such as wild sockeye salmon (Coho is sometimes farm raised), wild halibut, wild sable, wild Dover sole, walnuts, and pumpkin seeds. Second, the absence of processed foods, grains, and frying techniques will reduce saturated fat sources to reasonable levels. Trans fats need to be eliminated completely. Cheese, butter, and dairy fats should be used sparingly, but frankly are not ideal.

Beef intake should be low, and processed meats eliminated, because they create insulin surges and function as high-GL foods. Processed meats such as sausage, bacon, pepperoni, and almost all lunchmeats are unhealthy for you.

Fat can be an innocent filler in your diet, as you shift away from sugar. Remember that **sugar (carbohydrate) is the fuse that lights the fat bomb**. If one does not provide the fuse, one cannot ignite the bomb.

Protein

Very satisfying and safe macronutrient

Proteins are comprised of a sequence of amino acids. Humans have 20 amino acids. Nine are essential—not synthesized by the body. Eleven are nonessential. Three cannot be made in any way (from precursors or otherwise) and can be referred to as metabolically required: lysine, threonine and tryptophan.

Protein requirements

Protein dietary needs change depending on the age of the patient, co-existing pathologies, and exercise patterns. The more you exercise, including aerobic long duration exercise, the more protein you need. It is a common misconception that long distance athletes do not need as much protein as other more anaerobic athletes. In fact, many elite long distance athletes require more protein intake because of muscle breakdown from their long distance activities. The more muscle mass you have, the more protein intake is needed to maintain it. Below, we discuss the guidelines that describe the amount of protein intake that is suggested, and why the upper limits of protein intake have been increased.

Minimum & safe protein in sedentary adults

The minimum required protein intake for humans is 0.66 g/kg or about 0.3 g/lb. This is the minimum amount of quality protein that should be eaten by a non-active adult. So, if you are 30 years old and weigh 160 pounds, your minimum protein intake is 48 g, which is about 12 ounces of chicken breast (pre-cooked weight). Most chicken breasts are around 6 ounces, so figure on at least 2 chicken breasts. If you eat less, you are likely to lose lean muscle.

This is not the amount of protein a person who exercises, trains, or is growing needs. Such people need more protein to build musculoskeletal support.

Protein quality and disease risks

Quality protein (lean and wild) is very healthy and safe

Although your protein intake requirement increases as you age, we strongly suggest diets focused on quality protein sources; *always including unprocessed foods* and sources such as wild-caught coldwater fish and properly raised poultry. In the aging population, grain-fed red meat confers little to no benefit over other protein sources.

Like with bone, muscle is constantly reshaping. This leads to what we call *turnover*. Think of shaping a clay sculpture. You will regularly remove and add back pieces to shape your product. The body does the same with bone and muscle, though with bone it is slower. Proteins are removed and added back to muscle daily. As we age, this process increases, with the removal phase starting to play a more dominant role; after all, we are decaying. Additionally, as with all systems, the efficiency of replacing the protein is diminished. For these reasons, we need more protein when elderly (>65 years old) than we did in our middle-aged years (45–65).

The biological value of animal vs. plant protein is often debated, and might be for some time to come. As we have with carbs and fats, new studies need to be more specific about what proteins (amino acids), and from what source, cause or are correlated with what outcomes. Right now, the broad variety of proteins used in studies makes it difficult to be conclusive about the health value of plant vs. animal proteins. Below is a review of what we do know.

Net use of protein from animal sources approaches or equals 1, which is perfect. Studying protein use in children is a little easier than studying it in adults. Children clearly benefit from animal protein because of its near perfect balance. With adults, the evidence is not as clear. In large part, the amount of nonessential amino acids eaten will determine the need for the essential amino acids (found more substantially in animal proteins). The more nonessential amino acids eaten, the less need for essential amino acids.

On balance, if lean wild fish and poultry are your source of protein, you will more likely be getting higher quality protein than from vegetable sources.

It is important to keep in mind that the quality of any product (animal or vegetable) is related to the quality of what it was fed. Thus, if it is fed healthy food, it will be healthier. We know this to be true by analyzing the nutrient value of different food products that are fed different diets. For example, it is well established that grain-fed beef is more inflammatory and less healthy than grass-fed beef. The same can be said for people, as we now know. "Carb-fed" people will have more body fat than "lean protein-fed" people.

Protein and cardiovascular disease risk

Wild-caught high protein diets will reduce your risk of heart disease

Wild-caught fish and poultry (or game) will reduce heart disease risk. Free-range lean cuts (breast meat) of farmed poultry is also heart healthy. However, heart disease risk is increased with grain-fed red meat consumption, especially *processed* grain-fed red meats. We know that for each serving of grain-fed beef:

- Unprocessed grain-fed red meat increased risk of heart disease by 18%.
- Processed grain-fed red meats risk of increased risk of heart disease by 21%.
- Risk of dying from heart disease was increased by 13% for each 3 oz. serving of unprocessed grain-fed red meat.

We also know that low-GL and high-protein content diets result in lower heart disease. We know that patients who reduce carbs to 34% and raise protein intake to 24% (well within safe amounts), have half the heart disease risk as those who have carb intake at 45% and protein intake at 14%.

In short, higher carbohydrate diets lead to proportionately higher risk of heart disease, whereas higher protein diets are associated with leaner bodies, less fat, and less risk of heart disease.

Protein and cancer risk

Stay away from processed meats, grain-fed beef, and excess grilling.

We know cancer risk is increased with grain-fed red meat consumption, especially processed grain-fed red meats. The risk of cancer related death is about 10% more for those who eat more red meat than those who do not. And the risk of cancer-related death is about 16% more for those who eat more *processed* red meat than others.

High-temperature grilled grain-fed red meat also increases the risk for certain cancers. Grilling produces carcinogens such as aromatic hydrocarbons and heterocyclic amines.

Aging patients are advised to substantially reduce grain-fed red meat to infrequent consumption—less than a single 3 oz. serving per week. Grass-fed beef is higher in omega-3 fatty acids and is leaner than grain-fed. Nevertheless, infrequent consumption is still advised for grass-fed beef as well.

In short, grain-fed red meat and all processed meats are unhealthy. The risk of cancer is higher in those people who eat more grain-fed red meat, but it is not necessarily a causative relationship. Often, those who eat grain-fed red meat have other lifestyle habits that might be more contributory to developing cancer.

Protein and DMII risk

Unless it is processed meat or grain-fed beef, higher protein diets will likely reduce your diabetes risk

We can observe in the lab and through experiments that amino acids can cause insulin levels to rise, and grain-fed red meat is associated with risk of diabetes. We have not shown that varying the protein macronutrient mix (increasing protein intake for example) changes the risk of DMII. We have experiments that show increased protein diets do not increase the risk of diabetes.

In contrast to protein, however, we have shown that reducing the GL and sugar intake does reduce the risk of DMII.

In short, some amino acids that make up proteins can contribute to insulin elevation. However, there is no evidence to suggest elevated protein in your diet contributes to risk of DMII. On the contrary, higher protein diets are associated with leaner bodies, less fat, and less risk of DMII.

Protein and osteoporosis

High-protein diets do not contribute to osteoporosis

Are high acid/high protein diets unhealthy? No

Whether high protein diets contribute to osteoporosis is quite controversial. Some researchers have shown animal protein intake results in lower bone mineral density (BMD), whereas others have shown animal protein intake increases BMD.

The theoretical mechanism (not proven despite attempts to do so) for protein contributing to reduced BMD (osteopenia early, osteoporosis later) has to do with the pH implications of diets with different macronutrient mixes.

> ***A diet high in grains or animal proteins tends to be more acidic because of phosphates and amino acids that contain sulfur. Vegetables and many fruits tend to be more alkaline because of the calcium, magnesium, and potassium.***

A lower pH is more acidic; a higher pH is more basic. H+ ions are acidic and HCO3- (bicarbonate) ions are alkaline (basic). Perfectly neutral, not acidic and not basic, is a pH of 7.0.

In general, the typical diet (in the USA) tends to be of a lower pH (more acidic). It is implied that eating acidic food creates an acidic environment in the blood. Normal blood pH ranges from 7.35 to 7.45, slightly alkaline. We balance pH in the blood largely by the kidneys excreting the acid (an H+ ion).

As we age, our kidneys are less efficient at removing acid from the blood and excreting it. This means that our bodies have to find another way to balance the pH, to make it more alkaline.

We know calcium can increase pH. Calcium comes from vegetables, but calcium can also be released from the bones when the pH is too low (acidic). Therefore, proponents of diet-induced osteoporosis, suggest that a more acidic diet, especially in the elderly, requires more calcium loss from bone to make sure the blood stays between 7.35-7.45 pH.

As clear as the diet/pH discussion might seem, there is little evidence to support reduction in BMD because of dietary intake. In part, this can be due to compensation of better calcium resorption in the small intestine with high protein diets.

In short, neither high acid nor high protein diets have been shown to increase risk of osteoporosis.

Does salt intake affect osteoporosis risk?

Salt does not change osteoporotic risk

As an exception, if a patient has a specific variation of a gene (polymorphism) that encodes the information for the vitamin D receptor, that patient is at risk for bone mineral loss (resorption). Such patients on higher salt diets (about 4 g/day) showed 25% more urine excretion of molecules that are known to reflect bone resorption and therefore a tendency toward reduced BMD. This is not true for people with the normal vitamin D receptor gene.

Therefore, as an exception, salt intake might affect osteoporosis risk in those with the genetic variation of the vitamin D receptor gene.

The lifestyle factors that impact protein choices such as resistance training, sun exposure to promote sufficient vitamin D, and intake of calcium from green leafy vegetables is more important for bone health that manipulating protein intake.

Whatever theoretical or practical effect protein has on bone turnover is negligible compared with the benefits of resistance training, higher protein, and lower GL diets. Dietary intake of vitamin D, calcium, bicarbonate, vegetables, and fruits can all ameliorate the acidic effects of high protein diets and high sodium diets.

Does high protein intake hurt your kidneys?

High protein intake does not hurt your kidneys if you have normal kidney function to start

In people with normal kidney function, high protein diets are not associated with harm to their kidneys. You can be sure you have no renal function impairment if you have normal lab values of kidney function. Your doctor can give you that information.

Does high protein intake lead to earlier death?

Controversial, but probably not. High protein intake protects against obesity.

In the case of saturated fats, we spent an enormous amount of resources to implicate saturated fat in premature heart disease. The effort was not wasted, because we found saturated fats are definitely NOT the cause of premature heart disease; rather, **it was lifestyle and other eating habits that often accompany those who eat more saturated fats in Western cultures.** We have discussed this at length in the section on saturated fats.

The studies associating mortality (and cancer rates) with increased protein intake are reminiscent of (and similar to) the first studies on saturated fats. Such studies are usually done with questionnaires that have limited detail and rely on the accuracy of the patient's memory. They are subject to many biases.

> ***It is likely, when a more in-depth and rigorous look at protein intake is made, that high protein diets will not be found to be a source of premature mortality or cancer; rather the source (red meats) and other habits that accompany middle-aged 'higher protein' intake, like eating burgers, fries, and rib eye steaks will be the culprit.***

Isn't that what most middle-aged 'high protein' diets are currently comprised of? None of the studies, to our knowledge, establish the clear source of the proteins and therefore the quality. The most specific studies we have seen divide protein sources into plant and animal, but animals come in many shapes and sizes. A lean halibut filet is much healthier than a grain-fed rib-eye steak and we are doubtful big fish and poultry eaters exhibit the same mortality rates as big steak eaters. Time will tell as the study qualities improve.

When should you use protein supplements?

Protein supplements have been shown to be beneficial before, during, and after exercise. If you have to choose one, be sure to take 30–40 g of mixed fast and slower absorbed protein supplements within 30 minutes of ending your workout, including after you go running.

Summary: Protein

Cut back on beef, and eat much more wild-caught fish

Mortality risk is well established to increase with *grain-fed* red meat consumption, especially *processed* grain-fed red meats. Processed meats include lunch meats, bacon, sausage, salami, and hot dogs. A serving of grain-fed red meat is 3 ounces or 85 g—about a fist size.

For each serving of unprocessed grain-fed red meat, risk of mortality increases by 13%; for processed grain-fed red meats, risk of mortality increases by 20%.

Protein intake with respect to mortality cannot be viewed in isolation. Intake in middle age is most likely a biomarker for other nutritional and non-nutritional habits that more directly influence health—such as processed and red meat consumption, sedentary lifestyle, alcohol intake, and smoking.

Summary: Macronutrients

Macronutrients include carbohydrates, fats, and proteins. They are the source of calories and they are messengers to metabolic and appetite systems (as we will see in the next section). They affect how food is managed in the body. Thus, you are what you do with what you eat.

Carbs are the fuse that lights the body fat bomb. Excess carbs lead to an insulin surge, which promotes fat building and prevents fat breakdown. Ultimately, carbs, not fats, are the cause of heart disease. Fat is implicated in heart disease after excess carbohydrates have led to blood vessel damage. Therefore, you want to eat carbs that do not increase insulin. We call those low GL carbs. They are found primarily in non-root vegetables. However, fruits have great benefits and are an excellent alternative to chips.

Fats (omega-3 fatty acids) can defuse the body fat bomb. Fats do not cause heart disease, but circulating cholesterol does increase the risk of heart disease if the vascular lining is already damaged from inflammation. Omega-3 fatty acids reduce inflammation, whereas omega-6 fatty acids increase inflammation. Eat foods with less omega-6 and more omega-3 fatty acids.

Protein is necessary to build the body. After 65 years of age, we are less efficient at processing protein, and therefore will require more. However, many people eat far less protein than they need to maintain their lean body mass. Unless you have compromised kidney function, high-protein diets (up to 35% of your total daily caloric intake) are very safe. Protein sources are typically given as precooked weight because how you cook the food influences the total nutritional value. We recommend a little butter when cooking, using baking and broiling as preferred methods. We often use herbs like turmeric and black pepper or other healthy herbs to add flavor. We use a rough guide of 1 ounce of animal meat (or egg) is about 6 g of protein. Chicken breasts range from 4–8 ounces, depending on size. Combining a low GL diet with high quality protein consistently improves body composition.

Severe caloric restriction is not recommended, although excess caloric intake is a root cause of obesity. Periodic fasting might be something to experiment with as you get comfortable with your body.

Appetite Regulation

Part IV

Introduction

*T*he decision to eat is more complex than you might consciously think. Food intake is regulated by two general methods, homeostasis and hedonics (and other non-homeostatic influences). We talk about what these words mean because they are important concepts in understanding how appetite is regulated.

Homeostasis is what comes naturally to the body. It is a way of balancing effects so that the net result is no or little change. Homeostasis is a general principle we see consistently throughout body systems—the body's tendency to keep things the same; balanced. We talked about bone turnover in the prior section, which is the tendency for the body to reshape the bone, slowly, adding and removing minerals but keeping the same bone density despite our diet or exercise routine changing. This is an example of homeostasis. With appetite, we see a tendency for the primitive part of the brain (hypothalamus) to regulate our food intake through hormones and other molecules, such that we tend to stay the same weight over a long period of time. The other way food intake and appetite are regulated is through the more conscious parts of our brain (frontal cortex) and their connection to the primitive parts. We can override the body's homeostatic tendency to stay in balance by using our frontal cortex. The frontal cortex can be a two-edged tool. We can deliberately override the body saying it is full, by choosing to eat the dessert, despite not being hungry. This type of food intake regulation is called hedonic appetite regulation. The word hedonistic means "engaged in the pursuit of pleasure." Thus, hedonic appetite regulation applies to the type of eating most of us do that gets us into the obesity zone. We might eat for comfort, stress management, or simply because the chips are so delicious we cannot eat just one. The upside is that the frontal cortex can be used to say "no," but it is harder than saying "yes." That is one reason we observe it is easier to gain weight than to lose it.

Today, the overabundance of foods is often in the form of processed food, which means they have atypically high calories, are unusually tasty or palatable, and sadly, are lacking nutritional substance. The hedonic mechanisms are usually the drivers of our contemporary eating habits. They need to be reined in, and the only way to do that is to use our executive function (frontal cortex of our brain) to say "no" more often. Because the topic of hedonics naturally raises the question of how appetite and drug addiction might have overlapping neuro-circuitry, we address this issue as well.

Hedonics

Pleasure-driven eating

In modern society, many people can afford the luxury of liking, or the pursuit of hedonic drives—including eating food just because it tastes great. Food is one of life's greatest pleasures, no doubt. Which is why it boggles the mind that people spend time eating a lot of really bad processed food. Hopefully, as you read and reshape how you see the foods you eat, you will realize that the compulsion to eat processed foods is not about enjoying the taste of the food. Processed foods exploit your dopaminergic system's drive for pleasure. Your brain is hijacked with processed foods. In the pursuit of a fulfilling life, we would say that balancing all of life's pleasures allows for a maximum net experience of pleasure. By focusing so much on food-derived pleasure, obesity robs many people of enjoying other pleasures in life. After all, if you are unable to enjoy a hike in the woods, the endorphins from a great workout, or being vigorous and amorous with your partner, your total pleasure in life is reduced to one domain: food. Checking your hedonic pleasure impulses for tasty food will probably allow for a much richer life experience. The hedonic drive we see today, combined with energy-dense, nutritionally depleted and overly palatable processed foods, contributes strongly to the epidemic of obesity. Without choosing actively and consciously to not eat, it is perfectly predictable that we will get fat.

We will review the specifics of homeostatic appetite control, looking especially closely at macronutrients and how they influence appetite beyond just being calorie sources. We will also review the specifics of non-homeostatic drives (including hedonics) and how they disrupt the homeostatic mechanisms of appetite control. Where molecular science merges with behavioral science, we will present the evidence that supports hedonic theories, closely related to the reward circuitry/systems of the brain. There is overlap with eating and addiction, but more importantly, there are substantial differences. We will discuss both the differences and the similarities.

Homeostatic Mechanisms of Appetite Regulation

Need-driven eating to keep energy systems stable

Physiological *needs* drive us to maintain a homeostatic energy state, reflected in the remarkably constant weight people tend to maintain without deliberate effort. The body usually attempts to defend or maintain a set weight point. How is that?

In part, the hypothalamus uses the total energy consumed to regulate appetite. Specific features of macronutrients also play a role in regulating food intake, as we alluded earlier to the fact that they not only contain calories, but also send signals that influence metabolism. Two additional factors influence weight maintenance: the volume of food eaten and the ability to compensate for the atrophy of muscle (which occurs as we use it less and less) with accumulation of body fat (body composition can change to keep your weight constant).

Homeostatic appetite control: The defended set point

Your body likes things to stay the same, which is one of the reasons it is hard to lose weight (body fat)

Body weight is closely controlled, or defended, as we know from observing our own lives. Our weight doesn't change much before middle age, regardless of how much time we take to think about what we eat. Our weight just happens to stay the same.

We also know it is easier to gain weight than to lose it. This makes sense from an evolutionary perspective and is put forward formally in the "thrifty gene theory" that suggests that periodic famines created pressure on gene selection for an organism that was more efficient. Gaining weight and making it hard to lose was more efficient than being able to quickly lose the weight. Also, the selection pressure for a more nimble and leaner organism was higher before shelter, fire, and weapons. As this pressure lessened over time, the pressure to stay lean was reduced. Now, we just have no reason to be lean, except for health purposes.

To a lesser degree, our bodies use the volume of food intake in defending the set weight point. Before processed foods, which pack an unnatural amount of energy into small volumes, this mechanism served us well. A balance of meat, vegetables, and other available foods, in general, yielded a relatively narrow range of calories per volume, even though eggs and kale can be considerably different in volume per calorie (calorie density). They are still closer in volume than the amount of calories you will find in a burger and fries.

Processed food makes eating tons of calories too easy. Today, we can shove a pint of ice cream into our stomachs in under an hour.

A pound of nuts, on average, is low in volume and highly dense in calories. In nature, a pound of nuts requires a lot more energy to collect, if you could even find them all ready to eat at the same time. Therefore, the volume contribution of maintaining a set weight point is not working so well today. Since the food industry started processing foods, it got even worse. When low-fat was the new craze, they packed foods with tons of sugar to make them palatable, increasing caloric density.

Evidence also suggests that the way the body maintains a set weight point is partly through altering body composition. Body composition is essentially comprised of fat and nonfat tissue (lean tissue such as muscle and bone). We discuss this more in detail in the exercise section. However, the bottom line is that a pound of fat takes up much more space than a pound of muscle. So, what happens in middle age? Our whole body metabolism slows and muscle atrophies. The body's propensity to maintain a set weight point means that as the lean mass decreases, the body fat increases. The increase in body fat (replacing the lost weight of atrophied muscle) shows up as love handles. The solution: reduce body fat by eating properly (much fewer carbs) and maintaining your muscle mass (with resistance exercises).

The hypothalamus is the appetite control center of the primitive brain

If you let it run the show, you will not likely get fat

The brain has critical centers that control appetite and energy metabolism. Specifically, the primitive parts of the brain, including the hypothalamus, are critical to this role, as are the hormones that act on it: ghrelin, leptin, and insulin

We have heard a lot about insulin already and know that insulin surges promote inflammation, body fat production, and inability to use fat as fuel. Ghrelin is best thought of as a stimulant to appetite. It is made in the stomach. When it goes up, you get hungry. Ghrelin acts much like someone might on a long car trip. The longer it's been since we last filled up, the more often they suggest we stop at the next gas station. When it has been quite some time and the low fuel alarm goes off, they start insisting you pull over at the next exit that has a station.

> ***Leptin is a hormone that is best thought of as a fuel gauge.***

Leptin is made in fat cells, and essentially tells your brain how full the tank is. As body fat rises, the fuel gauge moves toward full and you reduce the need to eat. Conversely, when you lose body fat, the low fuel alarm goes off, and the brain tells the body to "fill up." Leptin influences appetite by acting on the primitive brain when we fill up our fat cells. Say, for example, we have a 16 gallon-tank, but have 4 gallons of fuel in it. The signal will be to add 12 more gallons. The primitive brain has receptors to leptin. As with any receptor, they have a certain level of sensitivity. The more sensitive the receptors, the sooner you will stop filling up the gas tank. Leptin influences that degree of sensitivity of the brain receptors to the "stop, that's enough gas for right now" signal. That signal comes from hormones released in the small intestine during a meal. They influence how much we eat at one time. That is called satiation—the point in time where you experience a sense of fullness that tells you to put down the fork.

We know that chronic low levels of inflammation interfere with leptin acting on the hypothalamus. In a way, you can think of inflammation causing the fuel gauge to get stuck at a lower level—making you think you need to refill (eat), more than you really do. Chronic low levels of inflammation make receptors less sensitive to the "stop" signal on meal size, as well as reducing how much leptin actually gets into the brain.

Inflammation directly interferes with leptin's ability to tell the hypothalamus that the gas tank is full. This state of reduced amount of, and sensitivity to, leptin in the hypothalamus is called "leptin resistance."

In this state, we keep filling the tank because we don't realize it is full. The overflow of gas would be the extra body fat we gain. The brain is reset to think it has a 24-gallon tank. Even if we manage to decrease leptin by burning a lot of gas (reduce body fat), every time we fill up, the brain still thinks it has a 24-gallon tank.

Over time, chronic low levels of inflammation in the hypothalamus are thought to result in a new 'set point' of weight. If we don't lower the inflammation of the hypothalamus and reset the brain back to its original set point of lower weight, relapse of the weight loss is likely, because the body still tries to defend the higher weight. This is one reason it is so hard to lose weight. It takes time and consistent effort to keep redirecting the hypothalamus until it finally understands a new set point is needed.

The defended set point is possibly the initiating event leading to diet-induced obesity. Excess calorie diets cause inflammation of the hypothalamus and contribute substantially to the leptin resistance seen in obese patients. Peripherally, such inflammation clearly contributes to insulin resistance. Thus, inflammation, both peripherally and centrally, is implicated in obesity.

Acute and long-term signaling occurs with eating. The acute changes reflect response to a current meal. The long-term signaling occurs primarily through insulin and fat cells (and their hormones), which reflect the long-term energy balance status. Homeostatic regulation tends to very tightly controlled, allowing for very stable weights over long-term periods of time, despite quite varied intake of calories. In most of us, the homeostatic metabolic system can be subservient to higher brain functions and hedonic drives. We can choose not to eat. However, many of us do not choose to exercise this capacity.

Macronutrients are not just calories, they also send signals to the brain that regulate appetite

Of the 3 macronutrients, carbs are the only non-essential one, which speaks to the lack of value carbs play in survival and health.

In an academic model that was created to assess behavior when one macronutrient was completely taken away, the following interesting results shed light on which macronutrients were most 'needed' and therefore sought if they were removed.

Protein

We tend to seek protein when it is low

Behavioral evidence defending a target protein level through regulated intake is strong. Mice have learned to avoid diets depleted of essential amino acids. Proteins also have the highest satiety factor of all of the macronutrients. In young growing animals, high-protein diets are sought.

Fats

We do not tend to seek dietary fat when it is low

In contrast to protein and carbohydrates, the academic model of macronutrients does not suggest that we prioritize fatty acids, even if they are the only source of energy remaining. This is not to say fat does not influence metabolism. It does. It is second to protein in promoting satiety. It simply means that if you remove fat from the diet, the preferred macronutrient source will never be fat, despite it being absent. Protein will be sought.

Carbohydrates

We do not tend to seek carbs unless they are very low

Behavioral evidence for defending a target carbohydrate level through regulated intake is weak (but not absent), despite all of the attraction to sweets we might exhibit. Nevertheless, an academic model suggests animals do eat toward a target carbohydrate level. Protein intake supersedes carbohydrate-seeking behavior, however. This might explain why a diet of <20 g is intolerable to almost everyone, but one of 50-100 g is quite tolerable, if not preferred, over the long term.

Summary: Homeostatic Mechanisms

You can maximize your body's natural tendency to keep to a specific weight by eating a diet of low-GL (low and slow carbs) and high protein. Better stated, we suggest you stop eating the high carb/low protein diet.

A protein diet of about 25% to 35% of all calories you eat is very safe and effective at optimizing muscle and minimizing body fat.

By reducing your GL for the carbs you eat (not more than 30% of all calories), you will maximize burning fat. You will also minimize inflammation.

The remaining 40% of your calories will come from fat. The fat sources will minimize inflammation in your body *if they are largely omega-3 fatty acids*, such as wild fish, lean poultry, and nuts.

> ***By minimizing inflammation you will reduce the tendency for your brain to become insensitive to the hormones that control your appetite.***

In particular, leptin stops working effectively in the brain, the fuel gauge that tells you when to stop refilling your tank and that tells your brain how big you fuel tank is. Inflammation in the brain stops leptin from telling you that you are full.

Hedonic and Other Means of Appetite Regulation

We know that homeostatic mechanisms for regulating appetite tend to keep our body weight, and to a lesser extent, body composition, remarkably stable over a long period of time.

Let's look at other influences on appetite and see how they can contribute to disruption of that natural tendency to keep weight stable. We will touch on the environmental influences of appetite and food intake, such as food timing and emotional stress, which can contribute significantly to weight gain. Then, we will discuss how hedonics drive the desire to eat, including the big differences and smaller similarities of appetite regulation compared with drug addiction.

Environment

Find like-minded people in the early stages of your program

Your environment has a substantial impact on food intake behavior, ranging from social cues to stress. Environmental cues are an enormous part of the obesity epidemic, which we have partially discussed regarding the situation of constantly available food and the lack of transparency in food packaging. It is our observation as well that a supportive home and work environment strongly increases the probability of success in a new program. People who have partners, or whole families, start a new program, or who have access to a good supportive clinical team, succeed more often.

Stress and mood disorders

Both are closely tied to eating disorders and weight gain

Emotional stress can be a significant contributor to weight gain. In rodent models, mice subjected to social defeat showed significant increases in ghrelin levels and corresponding weight increases because ghrelin increases your appetite. Control mice lacking ghrelin receptors did not gain weight. Yet the mice with increased ghrelin, regardless of receptor status, showed more depressive symptoms than those without ghrelin increase. Chronic stress is associated with decreased leptin, which means the period of time you are supposed to think your gas tank is full is shortened, causing you to think you need more gas than you do, so you refuel earlier.

Change in appetite is a central component to major depressive disorder. About one quarter of the people with obesity have a mood disorder, convincingly linking obesity with altered emotions. This is not to erroneously conclude that one causes the other. It is simply an observation that mood disorders and obesity are often found together.

Hedonics (the pleasure principle of food)

Rely less on food for pleasure. Allow for other sources of pleasure in your life.

The biggest hurdle we find in most patients trying to reduce body fat is the struggle with the impulse to eat. This is especially true in the past 100 years, since the birth of food processing in the grain then dairy industries. The problem accelerated when the food industry began processing other foods, competing for consumer taste buds and indirectly exploiting primitive drives. The final problem (we hope) has been the colossal misconception that dietary fats cause heart disease. That gave the misdirected food industry yet another weapon against the consumer. They removed fat, and added volumes of sugar to replace the lost 'tastiness' of the foods they processed. The foods became even higher in caloric density yet, were entirely unsatisfying (in contrast to foods that contain protein and fat). The result is what we have now: the global epidemic of obesity. So, let's examine this hedonic system on a biological level to see how it works.

Potent hormones of the hedonic system, including opioids, dopamine, and to a lesser extent, endocannabinoids and serotonin, are essential to the reward system. We are all familiar, at least in part, with those terms, right? Heroin, cocaine, and marijuana act on the opioid, dopamine, and endocannabinoid systems, respectively. Thus, at least superficially, validating what we discussed previously: the limited overlap of drug addiction with food intake.

The most abundant receptors involved in hedonics include mu-opioids and cannabinoids. Both primitive and cortical brain structures are implicated in hedonics. The cortical part gives us an element of control over the primitive system, if we let it. The choice you have to impose control over the impulse to eat is what we might call "willpower." Without it, you cannot stop the urge to eat. For some this comes easily, for others less so. And for those already insensitive to hormones (such as insulin and leptin) it can take more time to return to a new set point—recruiting your homeostatic mechanisms to help you resist eating more. Without your deliberate effort to limit food intake, your hedonic systems will try to seduce you. And today, the urges can be overwhelming with all of the packaged super tasty, super energy-dense (nutritionally depleted) processed foods constantly available.

Opioids reinforce the palatability of food, but their effects are lost with fasting. When opioid antagonists are present, palatability is diminished.

Endocannabinoids help maintain food intake, as many people in Colorado can attest. Reduced leptin sensitivity, which typically suppresses appetite or feeding action, leads to increased endocannabinoid levels. The peripheral systems, such as fat cells, also have endocannabinoid receptors, which promote fat production.

The clearest evidence that liking includes higher brain regions are from imaging studies that showed the feeling of pleasure, or liking something, is encoded in the medial orbitofrontal cortex. Thus, hedonics is controlled by conscious cortical and unconscious primitive brain impulses. The side that wins dictates whether you say yes or no to food when you aren't hungry.

Worsening hedonics: A contemporary problem of a primitive drive

Indulgence is only known as a contrast to restriction

Since the industrial revolution, significant and contributing factors play strongly into our hedonic pursuit of food intake. Readily available food makes eating convenient, so both size and frequency of meals is easily increased. Hourly movement has diminished with urbanization, automobiles, and more sedentary professions. The quality of food products has diminished, with higher energy density and higher toxicity. Toxicity manifests in two ways. First, more carcinogens and inflammatory chemicals are present in food. Second, palatability increases to abnormal levels by increased fat and sugar or sugar substitutes, creating a toxic effect resulting in addictive hedonic behaviors. Unfortunately, the hedonic drive combined with energy-dense, nutritionally depleted, and overly palatable food products contributes substantially to the epidemic of obesity. As we said very early in the chapter, we believe this is a much greater contributor to obesity than reduced hourly energy expenditure due to more sedentary work.

Furthermore, the modern world is filled with an overabundance of stimulation, compared with a century ago. Food intake is easily conditioned, even in the absence of metabolic need. Habits, such as eating and watching TV or eating and playing video games, can easily lead to unnecessary caloric intake.

To compound all of the above, neuromarketing has become an arguably unethical and inarguably powerful cue and stimulator for food intake, especially in children and adolescents. Neuromarketing is a relatively new but powerful field of marketing that studies the physiologic response of consumers to different stimuli. This allows the marketing agency to maximize the appeal and sale of a product. Essentially, neuromarketing is a field of marketing that exploits consumers' responses to cues that impact the cortical and primitive brain centers. The idea is to know what will make a consumer buy a product and use that knowledge to seduce the consumer into buying it through packaging and promises.

It seems such powerful neuromarketing would suit people's health optimally if it was used to target healthy food consumption rather than just promote hedonic circuit activation. Granted, in order for the food industry to benefit, they would have to change their model from pedaling poison to pedaling healthfulness.

Appetite and Addiction: Are There Parallels?

Yes, but the differences are greater

The idea that behavior associated with food intake, particularly in the obese, is similar to behavior of drug addicts is a common parallel drawn in the health care industry. There are overlaps, to be sure. But there are significant differences, which are important to keep in mind as you manage your appetite. In all probability, there are probably "addiction" circuitry overlaps with all behaviors that compel us, ranging from iPhone use to exercise habits.

Evolutionarily, drug addiction is much newer than controls for energy and nutrient intake, so it seems plausible a more integrated system exists for controlling food intake than for controlling drug intake. The system for controlling food intake involves nearly all levels of endocrine- and neurocircuitry, so it is not surprising there is overlap with addiction.

Below we highlight the differences and similarities between eating and drug addiction. We start with the differences because we believe they are more important than the similarities and offer a place to start in changing behavior. We provide the similarities to help you understand that your belief that something is compelling you to make irrational choices of eating habits is founded in reality. You are right, there are forces at work that create a tendency to eat the wrong thing and even too much of a good thing. The rational conclusion is that you have to create an environment or setting where exercising self-control is possible, if not probable.

Differences between appetite and addiction

Initiating Event

- Drug intake starts with a pharmacological event, eating does not.
- Drug addiction is associated with depletion of dopamine in the nucleus accumbens of the hypothalamus. Food consumption is not.
- Dopamine activation is required for drug addiction. Eating might or might not be associated with dopamine activation (but not depletion).
- Drug addiction is strongly related to the central nervous system and is not substantially influenced by peripheral systems. Eating is strongly influenced by the peripheral nervous system, and appetite is regulated through the central nervous system. In fact, many of the molecules we eat contain not just calories, but send signals through the vagus nerve (an extensive cranial nerve) to the brain.
- Hormones that regulate eating also regulate metabolism, in a complementary way. For example, the "gas gauge" for eating is regulated by leptin, contributing to the period of satiety. During the period after eating, leptin increases metabolism, helping to burn the calories you eat and reducing the sense of hunger. Such a dual system has never been described in drug addiction.

Figure 4.1

Compulsive Behavior

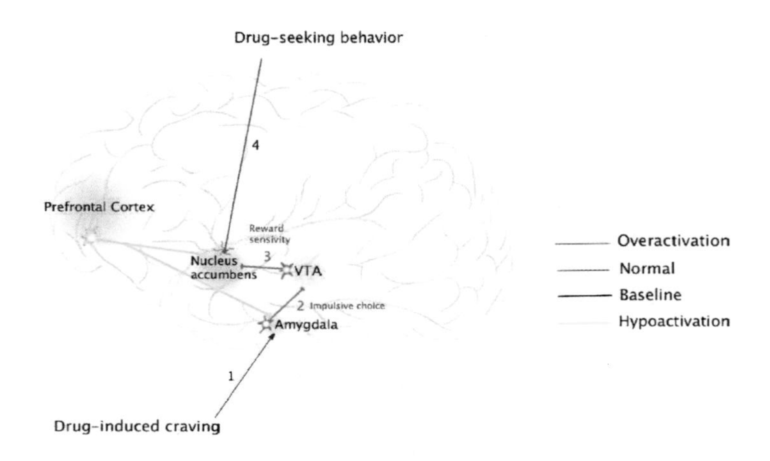

Similarities between drug pathways and appetite control

Brain centers

- The lateral hypothalamus in the brain contributes substantially to the reward system of drug abuse. It is also the brain's "hunger" center.
- Pre-signaling occurs where senses are engaged before the event. Pre-signaling is powerful in both drug abuse (habits and rituals before the event) and in eating. The amygdala-prefrontal-striatal circuitry has been shown to be active under both circumstances.
- The prefrontal cortex (PFC) helps regulate social behavior and decisions weighing risk and reward. It is what seems to be lacking in our teenage children. Drug addiction is associated with deficits in the prefrontal cortex. With food, an increase in PFC activity occurs with sugars (through μ opioid receptors). Fats and processed foods have both been associated with molecular changes in the PFC. Patients with frontal lobe dementias (not Alzheimers) eat more. They show less deliberate restraint in controlling the impulse to eat.

Neuropeptides

- Neuropeptide Y (NPY) stimulates both food and drug intake.

Observed behavior

- High fat, high carbohydrate, and processed food diets elicit irrational behavior, despite an increase in body fat and all that comes with obesity. Drug addiction also elicits addictive behavior, despite negative consequences.
- Reinforcement behavior is seen strongly with drug addiction and less strongly with eating.

It is no surprise there are some overlapping pathways of addiction and eating. The overlap is largely a reflection of how deeply integrated eating is to human existence, rather than a reflection of how closely it is related to drug addiction. Because eating involves the peripheral nervous system and the central nervous system, and has both homeostatic mechanisms and hedonic mechanisms that regulate it, it was bound to overlap with many things. Eating touches on virtually every system.

Summary: Appetite Regulation

Appetite is the drive to eat. Hormones are instrumental in regulating appetite. Insulin, leptin, ghrelin, and dopamine are strongly implicated in different pathways of appetite regulation.

Appetite is tightly regulated by homeostatic mechanisms driven by trying to maintain a balance between ingested and stored energy sources. Thus, energy balance is a balance between the types of calories we eat and how much fat we have stored. This balance is largely created through changing levels of hormones and results in a remarkably stable weight, in the absence of nonhomeostatic influences.

The types of foods we eat, not just the amount of calories, influence appetite. Different hormones respond when different types of foods are eaten. Thus, a calorie is not just a calorie. For example, sweet food can stimulate leptin secretion, which in turn reduces dopamine secretion, helping to control a “positive” response to sweet tastes, serving as a safety mechanism from overindulging in sweets. Mice who do not have this pathway are massively overweight.

Aside from the energy balance drive, appetite is also regulated by thoughts and emotions. In fact, the current obesity epidemic is a testimony to how thoughts and emotions can override homeostatic mechanisms of appetite drive. It is this component of nutrition that is often not addressed, and therefore leaves you and others frustrated with your effort to lose body fat.

Modernity has surpassed our evolutionary needs. Food is now constantly available—never in shortage in the Western world. Much of the food that is available is also abnormally high in calories and is excessively tasty, seducing us into eating more. Simply put, the more hands that touch our food, the less healthy it is. Many hands now touch our food between the farm and our mouth. You, as a sentient being, can take steps to deliberately eat what is good for you. Once you are in touch with your body, it will be easier to use a top-down approach to control overstimulated primitive brain impulses.

We must accept the bitter truth that we cannot simply consume food exclusively based upon hedonic drives, because most of what you think you want will kill you. We must eat based upon what we need—at least most of the time.

Food Planning

Part V

Introduction

A calorie is not just a calorie. We have touched on that truth several times, but now we are going to explain exactly why. Let's examine each macronutrient.

Why is a carb not just a carb? Low-GL carbohydrates do not contribute to elevated insulin and incretins. High-GL carbohydrates contribute to a less favorable heart disease risk profile, in part by reducing sensitivity to hormones like insulin and incretins and by promoting a pro-inflammatory state. As a whole, carbs promote fat accumulation and prevent fat from being used as energy.

Why is a fat not just a fat? Omega-3 fatty acids have anti-inflammatory properties and protective effects against heart disease. Omega-6 fatty acids promote inflammation. Both omega-3 and omega-6 fatty acids are essential fatty acids, and more specifically, both are PUFAs.

> ***Beware of universal comments about PUFAs—we now know that not all PUFAs are the same.***

Why is a protein not just a protein? Proteins are comprised of amino acids that vary in how they impact insulin secretion. Several amino acids are essential, whereas others are conditionally essential. Although individual amino acids can promote insulin secretion, the net effect of proteins as a macronutrient has generally little to no effect on insulin. They differ considerably from the insulin surges caused by carbohydrates.

Weight Loss

Weight loss = body fat loss. Less food intake is central to sustained weight loss.

When we discuss weight loss, we are really talking about body fat loss—nobody is avidly trying to lose muscle. In most people, we are even more specifically talking about visceral fat loss because it is the type of fat most closely tied to increased health risks, contributing the most to inflammation and heart disease.

Two major types of fat in adults are visceral adipose tissue and subcutaneous adipose tissue (SAT). Low testosterone levels are associated with VAT accumulation. VAT is more metabolically active and has more androgen receptors than SAT.

Macronutrient contribution to body fat loss

Lower carbohydrates = lower insulin surges that help you burn fat

As early as 1956, scientists realized that the mix of macronutrients was more important for predicting body fat or weight gain than a single macronutrient's caloric value. In a study assessing caloric intake at 90% of a single macronutrient, a diet of 90% fat predicted more weight loss than 90% protein or carbohydrate. Since that study, our understanding of the macronutrient mix has deepened. Thus, before the low-fat craze, we had studies that established a more positive relationship with macronutrient fat intake and body fat loss, relative to either carbohydrates or protein.

Yet, we went through decades of focusing on low-fat diets, in part due to the interest in reducing heart disease. Perhaps because heart disease risk factors include circulating lipoproteins that carry cholesterol, as a scientific community, we believed that lowering fat intake would reduce them. When fat intake was analyzed, saturated fats became the target because they do have a propensity to increase LDL—a known indirect risk factor for heart disease. Since those incorrect inferences, we have learned more about LDL and the overall impact of saturated fats. Now we know, as a group, saturated fats are not responsible for increased heart disease mortality rates. We also know LDL comes in several forms, one rich in TGs, which is dense, small, and a risk factor for heart disease; the other rich in cholesterol, big and fluffy, and not a risk factor for heart disease. So you see, not all LDLs are the same either.

Now we are focused on the role of carbohydrates and proteins in body fat management and heart disease risk and are trying to establish the appropriate macronutrient recommendations. In part, our recommendations might vary slightly, depending on your metabolic strengths and weaknesses, which are often reflected in laboratory values and through your history and physical. Below we examine different diets or food plans, primarily focusing on macronutrient mix differences.

How the low carbohydrate/high protein diet reduces weight

- *Protein costs more energy to digest*
- *Protein signals the brain that you are full*

We know protein-rich diets lengthen the time that you feel full, which leads to reduced food intake. There are two main reasons why we see weight loss with high protein diets, and it isn't because the food is so bad we don't want to eat it. The first has to do with the cost of energy needed to generate needed sugar from the small intestine. Typically, the liver takes care of making glucose, but the small intestine contributes a significant amount when carbs are cut down in the diet, so the liver makes less. The second is that the glucose molecule that comes from the small intestine (by the portal vein), sends a signal to the brain (via the vagus nerve) which serves to fill up the fuel tank by increasing leptin. Therefore, you don't feel hungry because the gas gauge says you aren't low yet.

Dispelling the myth about clogged arteries causing heart attacks

High carbs cause heart attacks

Let's review what elevated insulin does and at the same time explain why clogged arteries is the wrong model of heart disease. Then, we will show how you can improve insulin sensitivity by changing your macronutrient mix.

Elevated insulin decreases fat breakdown and increases fat building, resulting in increased TGs, which store energy as fat. A TG has 3 fatty acids on a glycerol backbone. Those fatty acids are created with insulin surges.

As you know, TGs and cholesterol need to be carried in the bloodstream by lipoprotein particles (VLDL, LDL, HDL), similar to the example of the minibus. The riders are the cholesterol and TGs, and the minibus is the lipoprotein. When TGs are in excess, more minibuses are needed to carry them and the cholesterol. Unfortunately, when serious and dense TGs sit on the minibus, they squeeze out the more light hearted and buoyant cholesterol. The TG-rich minibus becomes denser but a bit unwieldy so the body chops it into still smaller minibuses. Cholesterol still needs a minibus to ride on, so the liver makes more minibuses (lipoproteins). The result is more numerous and more dense lipoproteins. Dense lipoproteins are the most likely to contribute to plaque formation, provided they can find an already vulnerable and damaged blood vessel to land on.

Blood vessel damage is first caused by excess inflammation.

Without inflammation, blood vessels are smooth and not prone to plaque formation, even when there are more circulating dense damaging lipoproteins. The minibuses need a place to park to unleash their wrath. As long as the blood vessel is healthy, there is no place for them to promote the plaque formation. There are no places to park, and they must simply keep driving around.

This explains why some patients with high numbers of dense damaging lipoproteins do not get heart attacks: they don't have damaged blood vessels. If they did, they would actually be more likely to have a heart attack. On the other hand, this also explains why most people with heart attacks do not have high levels of lipoproteins (LDL and others). Most people do have inflammation-damaged blood vessels. So even with normal lipoprotein levels, they have plaques form, which are the basis of heart attacks. In a way, you can think of the probability of a heart attack as a combination of the number of circulating lipoproteins *and* the amount of damage your blood vessels has sustained.

You see, both damaged blood vessels and damaging circulating lipoproteins are necessary for heart attacks. Carbs cause both. They cause damage to the blood vessel lining through elevated blood sugar levels, insulin surges, and inflammation. The insulin represses fat breakdown and promotes fat building, with excess circulating TGs.

Tips on weight loss

- You must want to lose body fat.
- It is ideal to objectively confirm weight loss is needed for your improved health. A DXA scan is ideal, because it quantifies the fat, shows where it is, and can be used to consistently follow progress.
- Identify prior efforts and barriers to success. If you have been successful before, but regained body fat, identify when the regain occurred relative to the loss. Plateaus in body fat loss are common and are to be expected. We often see a plateau at 6–8 months, then again at 1 year. If body fat reduction can be sustained at two years, we consider that a long-term success.
- Any plan should start out with success. The initial month's success or failure strongly predicts the 12-month sustained weight loss (or lack thereof). So, whatever plan you create, commit to it with 100% compliance for the first month. This is the only time where perfect execution is really useful. It is better to execute an imperfect plan perfectly than a perfect plan that fails. You and your care provider will help you make that plan. There is an overabundance of perfect plans out there, finding the best one is why you work with a team.
- We ask patients to come into a first visit with a week-long food diary that will help us identify low-hanging fruit, which includes tossing all items containing simple sugars, especially drinks. Once you start carefully reading labels, processed foods will start to fade, paving the way for a conversation highlighting the value of making your own meals. Avoiding the center aisles of prepared foods—shopping largely or exclusively in the peripheral aisles with fresh fruit and vegetables, lean meats and fish—is good simple advice. We also emphasize water before meals (improves satiation) and higher fiber diets, which paves the way for a whole food diet.

- Order your own food at restaurants. Request your own meals, even if not on the menu. Eating out does not have to be a nuclear bomb to your food plan, though it often is. Most restaurants will accommodate simply cooked orders such as grilled chicken and steamed vegetables. They will not usually put that on the menu, but they can make it very easily. The veggies might not be GMO-free, local or organic, and the chicken might have been grown in a pen, but relative to the burger and fries, or pasta with alfredo sauce, the grilled chicken and steamed vegetables will be much less damaging.
- Learn to cook food you like. It will save you money and unknown risks of eating out. It will also allow you to plan your daily meals better, which goes a long way toward sticking with your program.

Handy **portion control** advice includes the following:

Shorthand

Fist=1 cup
Open cupped hand= ½ cup
Flat palm = about 3 oz. of chicken or fish
Thumb volume = 1 teaspoon (useful for those who use salad dressing)

5210 rule

5 servings of vegetables
2 hours max bluescreen entertainment time (TV, movies, computer)
1 hour exercise per day—we discuss how useful exercise is later
0 simple sugars (soda, sugar in coffee, ditch all processed foods)

Summary: Weight Loss

The most effective nutritional plan for weight loss has two basic requirements. First, a caloric deficit must be created. Fewer calories must be taken in than are used. This is not to imply exercise will be central to losing weight. It won't. The idea is to focus on eating less.

The second requirement is a high degree of compliance. Studies clearly show weight loss comes with consistent effort, not short-term suffering. Do something you can do and can continue doing.

Although we advocate a low-carbohydrate approach as the first and best plan, we recognize any sound plan that can achieve a calorie deficit.

A well periodized exercise program facilitates efforts in body fat reduction, and should be an integral part of any plan. However, exercise will not be the major force in reducing body fat. We talk about what a periodized exercise program is in the chapter on *Exercise*.

Short-Term and Popular Diet/Food Plans

Pick what works for you and stick to it for a month. They have similar results.

Innumerable food plans and other nearly perfect (and vastly imperfect) dietary recommendations exist. Developing your own, with the guidance of a successful team, is the best approach. Each person is substantially different in how they deal with appetite regulation from an emotional level and how they deal with stress. There is less variation in the way people metabolize food, though a small amount of variation exists, as highlighted by APOε gene variations and response to dietary carb intake, as we have already discussed.

Most initial shortcomings in weight control have nothing to do with physiology, though bad eating habits can create bad physiology over extended periods.

Which diet works best for improving health markers?

- *Effects on cholesterol:* High soluble fiber diets (>30 g) reduce cholesterol most effectively. This is often captured in the anti-inflammatory diet plans.
- *Effects on insulin:* High-protein diets result in better insulin sensitivity.
- *Effects on leptin (the appetite fuel gauge):* Low GL diets result in better leptin sensitivity
- *Gender trends:* Women tend to lose weight more slowly, possibly due to differences in postprandial (the period after a meal)

glucose and fat oxidation. For weight loss and reduction of TGs in women, reducing the GL is more important than it is for men. Women show higher increases in total cholesterol than men. Women also respond with more substantial weight loss with the high protein diet, than other diets.

Which diets do people stick with the best?

The standard unhealthy diet and one that resembles a Mediterranean diet

Choosing a sustainable diet is the most important factor in long-term weight reduction and maintenance.

The two diet types that show the highest compliance are the typical anti-inflammatory diet (15% protein, 55% carb, with low GL) and the high protein diet (25% protein, 45% carb, high-GL).

The high-protein anti-inflammatory diet (25% protein, 45% carb and low-GL) and typical diet (15% protein, 55% carb, high-GL) are least adhered to, but the low-GL diets have substantial health benefits.

Which diets help reduce DMII?

The low carb/high protein and Mediterranean diets

The two diet plans described above resulted in the most substantial lowering of leptin levels. As we know from the section on *Appetite Regulation*, leptin resistance is strongly linked to whole body insulin insensitivity. Leptin resistance is well documented in obesity, and is implicated in insulin resistance and DMII. The observation that the two favored diets resulted in the most substantial reduction in leptin levels suggests those diets likely improve insulin sensitivity. Improved insulin sensitivity means lower risk for DMII.

> ***As a long-term marker of health on multiple levels, preserving or restoring insulin sensitivity is one of the most critical parameters.***

Which diets help reduce heart disease?

Low carb/high protein diets

The *most healthy diet is the high protein diet.* It has the most favorable impact on the ratio of HDL to total cholesterol. The second-most favorable diet was the typical anti-inflammatory diet. It has the most fiber and most favorable impact on total cholesterol.

Summary of macronutrient effects on short-term body fat loss

Protein

High protein and low-GL food plans give you the most body fat loss. Reducing GL requires a strong shift toward non-white vegetables, with few fruits while eliminating grains (crackers, bread, rice, cereal, quinoa). Higher protein diets tend to have *lower* GL, by nature of reducing carbs to allow for the increase in protein.

Carbohydrates

Lower GL diets are associated with body fat loss.

Fats

Dietary fat intake is not correlated with weight loss.

Fiber

High soluble fiber (30 g/day) diets are shown to significantly reduce LDL and total cholesterol. In part, this might be related to the low GL diets.

Long-term weight maintenance

Long-term weight maintenance is best achieved with consistent total caloric intake, balanced by exercise programs and proper sleep**.** The food plans with varying macronutrient mixes have no significantly different impact on weight. Therefore, once you are at the weight you want, eat what mix of macronutrients you wish to maintain that weight. Keep in mind, it is still healthier to eat low-GL, regardless of weight.

Mediterranean

Vegetables are a primary source of carbohydrates and dietary fats in the Mediterranean diet. It has high compliance, perhaps because it allows for all food groups (except dairy and meat which are strongly limited). It is an excellent alternative to low-GL/high-protein diets if you find them intolerable in the long term.

Atkins

The Atkins diet can be an effective approach for short-term, highly-motivated patients who plan to transition into a more sustainable food plan. It has a very low compliance over time and because of the low fiber, might not be healthy in the long term.

Zone diet

The Zone diet gets it right on two levels: reducing insulin surges and increasing the protein content of meals. The meal frequency has strong support in the bodybuilding community's experience, but is not supported in studies.

Weight Watchers

Weight Watchers is appealing because it allows you to choose what foods to eat and provides rough educational feedback on those choices. It encourages higher fiber content and reducing processed foods, which we believe are essential to long-term health. One of the less common features this program offers is a sense of community, which we believe encourages long-term participation.

Paleo

The Paleo diet is essentially a high-protein, low-carbohydrate diet without grains and legumes. It expresses a core principle of not eating processed foods, which might be its most valuable principle.

Ornish (Dean Ornish's Spectrum Diet)

Dr. Ornish was a pioneer in establishing that heart disease can be reversed by diet. One one hand it seems anything goes, but on the other hand, the diet is inordinately challenging to follow. A 10% fat diet is not something most people relish. The entire categorization process is subjective, making it uniquely Ornish, rooted only somewhat in science.

DASH (Dietary Approaches to Stop Hypertension)

The DASH diet was developed by governmental agencies, including the National Heart, Lung, and Blood Institute, thereby eliminating any chance of being on the mark. It is focused far too much on lowering salt, which has recently been shown to be misguided (similar to low-fat trends) and unsustainable. Furthermore, lowering salt, as we discuss later, is usually not needed for most patients. It still allows for 6–8 servings of grains, which is contrary to the advice from the results of most studies.

We recommend staying away from any government-sponsored programs on health and nutrition.

Safety and benefits of high protein diets

One of the most common questions we are asked by patients is whether or not a high-protein diet is safe. The short answer is that unless you have compromised renal function, YES a 35% protein diet is safe, as discussed in the previous section on *Macronutrients.*

Does it matter when or how often we eat?

Not really

For most of us, it probably does not matter when we eat. As we have said, our body has a way of regulating food intake over time. We do recommend a good breakfast, and minimizing eating within 2–3 hours of bedtime. But if calories and macronutrient composition are the same through the day, it probably does not matter whether they were spread out over 3 meals or 9 meals.

Cost of eating healthy (time and money)

- *Eating healthy is not a cost issue for most people*
- *Who pays for all of the ill health of unsound nutrition?*

The cost of eating healthy is $1.50 extra per day per person, according to a Harvard research study. Others argue that it is not any more expensive than traditional diets. We find that the more you cook at home, the seemingly more expensive healthy foods are not, over time, more costly than fast food, prepared foods, and processed foods, all of which incorporate into the price the cost of marketing and handling the food.

Patients often cite time as a factor for not preparing foods, but considerable amounts of time are wasted in lines, waiting for service, and paying for service. Keep that in mind when calculating the time it takes to cook your own meals. Foods can be very simple to prepare, and 2–3 meals can be prepared at a time, if necessary.

Finally, none of the cost estimates include the added cost of obesity, more frequent doctor visits, and other health care costs for bad nutrition (including a shorter lifespan of lower quality).

All things considered, the cost is almost certainly higher by not eating healthy. The question simply becomes how, when, and who will pay for the unhealthy choices.

Fasting

It's a good thing for a limited period of time

Fasting for variable periods of time has health benefits in otherwise healthy individuals. Restricted caloric intake, over a lifetime, is associated with a longer lifespan, but one can argue it creates a reduced quality of life. Such evaluations are very personal.

Other health benefits of intermittent fasting include an improved heart disease risk profile, decreased cancer risk, decreased DMII risk, improved cognition, decreased risk of Alzheimer's dementia and decreased risk of Parkinson's disease.

Reducing visceral adipose tissue

If you want to lose fat, that's where it's at

There is no definitive way to reduce VAT relative to other fat deposits throughout the body. But if there were a wonder drug to wish for, among others, it would be one that targeted the particularly unhealthy VAT.

The good news is that we do know of a few practices that *tend* to reduce VAT:

- Testosterone tends to reduce VAT.
- Timed whey protein intake of 20 g every three hours. Maximum effects of this approach are achieved when combined with exercise.
- Reduced alcohol intake. It seems alcohol goes directly to creating visceral fat.
- High intensity interval training—as is extensively discussed in the *Exercise* chapter.

Summary: Diets

Any plan, however well rooted in science that you cannot or will not execute is a failed plan. You will have to find a new one—one that you can execute consistently. Pick a plan, being 100% compliant for a month, then make adjustments that allow you to stick with most of the diet plan and still enjoy your food. Target a body fat level or weight loss goal and work with a team to get there. Along the way, you will learn a lot about your body. Once you arrive at your desired body composition or weight, you can adjust the macronutrient mix to your taste, but be vigilant about maintaining a caloric balance so you do not regain your hard-earned weight loss.

Summary: Food Planning

Today, nutrition is arguably the most important factor in the quality and longevity of life. While scientists strive to discover the amazing way the human body works and how it interacts with the environment, we are still a long way from healthfully manufacturing the nutritional value found in nature.

Ditch processed foods. They only add to the cost, and almost never improve a natural food product's healthfulness. The intersection of processed food and healthy food is essentially nil.

Food products are offered based on consumer demand. We currently demand tasty, convenient, long shelf-life food. Companies, by nature, are profit driven. Similar to the indifference of nature, companies are usually indifferent to whether their products or services have a positive or negative social impact. *Whole Foods* uses palm oil in their breakfast burritos. Profit allows a company to sustain itself, and is not a modifiable variable in the equation of food supply. Consumer demand is the only real modifiable variable.

Currently, consumer demand for highly palatable, energy-dense, but nutrient poor foods (processed food) outweighs consumer demand for healthy foods. Unfortunately, although the USDA might technically exist to safeguard the food supply, based on their history, it is not a reliable consumer advocate. At best, the government can be considered a null factor, but more realistically, they probably work more against the consumers' interests more than they protect the consumer.

Natural foods that are toxin-, hormone-, and antibiotic-free are central to a sound nutritional plan.

You are what your body does with what you eat (and what it ate or was fed). Animals raised in a drug-free, nontoxic wild or free-range atmosphere will produce healthier food products, both meat and milk. Although the products might look similar, nutritionally they are different. Animals, like people, are also what they eat. Food karma? The food industry's processing of foods, by definition will lead to less nutritional value and higher cost, even if caloric density increases because of processed sugars or other macronutrients. Processed foods are not a solution to global *nutritional deficiencies*, only caloric deficiencies. Processed foods will only contribute to higher health care costs. Not one example on the grocery store shelf can be found to the contrary.

Weight gain prevention starts with the awareness that the aging body is more susceptible to creating fat and prone toward harmful inflammation. Consider your 40s a decade to begin to improve your health, rather than giving in to the overwhelming tendency to deteriorate. It is the time when you are most likely to gain weight. Keep it off for that decade and you will be well on your way to aging well the next several decades.

Less caloric intake is required to prevent weight gain with age. Food intake must be reduced. Many factors work against appetite control, including a reduced need for calories with age, a genetic predisposition to store weight (especially in women), extraordinarily energy-dense but nutrient-poor processed foods that do not create proportionate fullness signals, easily accessible food products, and less fit and active people.

Many diets or approaches to food intake have been presented, with mild inter-diet variations of impact on body composition. Perhaps the most important lessons of food intake are the following:

A calorie is not just a calorie.

Each type of carbohydrate, fat, and protein can serve as signaling molecules to the body, producing nuanced but significantly different effects. For example, certain types of omega-3 fatty acids are anti-inflammatory and certain types of omega-6 fatty acids are pro-inflammatory, although both are essential fatty acids. Simple carbohydrates can elicit a significantly higher insulin response, whereas more complex carbohydrates can have a substantially lower insulin response, especially when consumed as a vegetable with high soluble fiber content. Some types of proteins elicit a strong insulin response, whereas others do not. So, a calorie is not just a calorie.

Fats, including saturated fats, are not a major contributor to heart disease. Carbohydrates are the culprit.

Carbohydrates contribute more to heart disease than any other macronutrient. Their contribution is largely inflammation-driven by increased insulin activity resulting in insulin resistance, higher circulating lipoproteins, and ultimately a higher probability of plaque formation.

Proteins, from whatever source, are satiating and drive small intestine gluconeogenesis; both of which contribute to reduced weight gain. Healthy functioning kidneys are not at risk for impaired function with high protein diets (35%). Protein sources (plant vs. animal) are controversial and will only be sorted out when controlled studies can specify what type of protein is eaten in what amount at what time.

Almost all people struggle with hedonic drives in appetite control because of the proximity and availability of food in general and processed foods especially. Some struggle more than others—they tend toward obesity. Thus, our current environment is *obesogenic*—it promotes obesity. The goal we have for you is to re-create a *leptogenic* environment that reduces obesity; the type of environment that existed, more or less, prior to processed foods. People who have long-term success begin to want what they need through a very slow change in values, perception of food, and behavior. The first steps in creating the leptogenic environment include surrounding yourself with other people of similar values and creating a first month plan to get your mind and body on track.

The complexity of appetite and weight loss is most substantially impacted by hedonic factors. Hedonics is also the most complex factor for us to help you with, but we can and do so successfully. We often see patients successfully apply the physiological benefits of appropriate energy balance and macronutrient choices during our induction phase, which is sort of like boot camp. During this phase, impressive results can be achieved. However, sustaining the results requires deliberate work and effective support. We believe you need a way to identify how much hedonics plays a role in your appetite regulation.

We cannot eat all of what we want. We have to eat what we need, more or less. But, you can start to want to what you need. It is an active process that includes changing your perception, values, and behavior. It starts with ditching processed foods.

Selected Topics

Part VI

Water

Drink more water, especially before meals.

There are many questions concerning how much water one should drink. For those who don't drink caffeinated beverages, the simplest approach to water balance is to have nearly clear urine, which indicates a well-hydrated state. Exercise, altitude, winter weather, and wind can all increase the need for fluids.

If you are urinating too frequently, you might want to cut back on your water intake and see how it changes your urine. If it is still nearly clear, you can stay with the lower amount.

For those of us who drink caffeinated beverages, which is not unhealthy in small to moderate amounts (<200 mg or approx. 2 cups per day), the urine after caffeine consumption will usually be nearly clear, even if you are mildly dehydrated. You should therefore rely on the end-of-day urine color, given that you probably quit drinking caffeine before 2 pm. For those of us who drink caffeine all the time, we suggest you address this issue with more urgency than the finer points of hydration. Excess caffeine interferes with sleep patterns, which can lead to long-term quality of life and longevity concerns.

Dairy: Is It Healthy?

Dairy includes milk, cheese, yogurt, and cream. Milk is best viewed as a source of sugar rather than as a source of protein.

Q: Is cow's milk bad for you?

A: Probably

In short, milk products from cows are not healthful and can be harmful, depending on your current health condition and individual metabolism. As with alcohol, we believe that the alleged benefits of milk can be achieved without the potential risk. The data on the health benefits of milk are quite controversial, and there is a strong agricultural interest in keeping milk consumption high. This factor, combined with the difficulty in assessing the effects of milk in isolation, leaves us skeptical of the quality of the studies that assert the health benefits of milk.

Q: Is goat milk better for you?

A: Somewhat

Goat milk more closely approximates human milk in consistency; however, do you know of any adult goat that suckles? Milk might not be unhealthy for everyone, but we believe there is more risk than benefit. We suggest eliminating milk for 8 weeks and see how that affects your digestion, inflammatory diseases and body fat composition, as well as the laboratory markers of heart disease and DMII. Your doctor can help arrange the lab tests.

Q: What about giving milk to growing teenagers?

A: Give them whole milk

Milk can be appropriate for teenagers and individuals who are highly focused on building muscle (such as certain athletes), because it has a very digestible and optimal protein mix of short-acting whey and long-acting casein. However, milk is best viewed as a source of sugar. For healthy patients (not diabetic), milk promotes higher levels of insulin. There are a few studies that suggest that people with diabetes could benefit from milk consumption, but their results might be partly due to improved eating habits.

These benefits apply to whole unprocessed milk, because its health benefits decrease once it is processed.

What is processed milk, pasteurization, homogenization and skimming?

Almost all the milk you drink, unless you live on or very near a farm, has been processed.

The healthful properties of milk are better preserved with less processing. Pasteurization (heating followed by cooling) is arguably healthful because it reduces the microbial burden inherent in milk. A number of authors have argued that processing detracts from healthful microbial activity and inactivates important milk enzymes such as phosphatase, lactase, and galactose, the latter of which contribute to the digestion of the respectively named sugars found in milk.

Phosphatase is useful for preventing the binding of calcium by phosphorus, which makes calcium more bioavailable. Without the inherent enzyme action in milk, the endocrine glands (pancreas) could be under stress to produce more enzymes. Authors have postulated that such stress can contribute to the development of DMII.

Pasteurization also inactivates lipases that would otherwise digest homogenized milk fat globules during the normal course of milk distribution and storage, thereby preventing the milk from going sour.

Cow's milk has larger fat globules than milk from sheep and goats, thereby forming the characteristic thick layer of cream at the top. Milk homogenization was first commercialized around 1919, using a process that employed high-pressure mixing of the otherwise insoluble fat with the rest of the milk product, effectively emulsifying the fat.

It has been argued that homogenization creates a film that protects xanthine oxidase (a compound involved in atherosclerotic disease) from being digested, effectively creating a liposome-like delivery vehicle for this compound. The case was therefore made that homogenization contributes to the increased prevalence of atherosclerosis. This theory has been effectively disproven on several fronts. One of the most compelling studies on animals and humans showed no increase in circulating xanthine oxidase after homogenized milk was ingested.

Another theory on the unhealthiness of milk that lacks support suggests that A_1 b-casein in cow's milk contributes to type 1 diabetes mellitus. In fact, A_1 b-casein does not contribute to diabetes mellitus.

Whole milk contains vitamins A and D, but when the fat is removed to produce skimmed milk, vitamins A and D are also removed. Milk processors add *synthesized* vitamins A and D, which a number of authors have suggested are toxic forms of the vitamins. Removal of the fat removes the healthy fats, which are then not replaced.

Bovine growth hormone used to increase milk production results in the presence of insulin-like growth factor 1 (IGF-1) in milk. IGF-1 survives all of the above processes and is absorbed into the bloodstream of milk drinkers. IGF-1 has been linked to malignancies, including breast and colon cancer.

Milk is allergenic and contributes to an increased use of infant tympanostomy tubes. A number of authors have argued that milk contributes to additional allergenic response in adults. This is partly supported by the fact that men with heart disease have been shown to have increased circulating antibodies to cow milk proteins.

Dairy insulinogenic properties: Are they unhealthy?

Uncertain

Skimmed milk has much of the original fat removed. From a macronutrient perspective, skimmed milk contains about 55% lactose carbohydrates, about 45% proteins, and <5% fat. In contrast, whole cow's milk contains about 50% fat, 20% protein and 30% lactose carbohydrates. Curiously, both skimmed and whole milk have a GL of 9.

Both skimmed milk and whole milk have strong insulinogenic properties. However, those properties are not due to lactose, or at least not isolated lactose. The isolated consumption of lactose and water elicits significantly less of an insulin response when compared with milk. A substance in milk, other than lactose, must therefore be contributing to the increased insulin response.

It is known that the essential amino acids leucine and isoleucine, in addition to tryptophan and glutamine, create an insulin surge (insulinogenic). Valine, lysine, and tyrosine have also been implicated as insulinogenic amino acids. Although it is tempting to assert that their insulinogenic character is responsible for the measured insulin indices of milk, the same proportion of these amino acids are found in beef, which elicits approximately 1/3 the insulin response of milk. The additive effects of sugars consumed with the insulinogenic amino acids are shown when beef is consumed with glucose.

However, it is possible that the insulinogenic effects of milk are attributable to unidentified factors and are not simply due to lactose combined with insulinogenic amino acids.

Do other dairy products cause insulin surges?

Yes, except cheese

All other dairy products, including ice cream, fermented products such as kefir, yogurt, and cottage cheese, are significantly insulinogenic.

Cheese is not insulinogenic and is comprised of fat and protein, with usually 0–2 g of carbohydrates.

Summary: Dairy

Dairy is not an essential constituent of meal plans and can have drawbacks for a subset of people who have particularly allergenic responses, and its consumption can cause insulin surges in anyone. In the case of allergies or discomfort, the choice to remove dairy from the meal plan becomes simple. Often, the only way to know is to remove milk from the diet entirely and then restore it if the results are inconclusive.

Drinking raw, unprocessed milk (particularly unpasteurized) might be dangerous simply because of the unknown travel, storage conditions, and shelf time. It might be prudent to simply avoid milk altogether.

All factors considered, viewing milk (and related products such as kefir and ice cream) as a source of carbs is the most useful way to understand how milk affects your food plan.

Osteoporosis: Calcium and Vitamin D

BMD begins to decline by age 30. The decline in BMD is partly slowed by estrogen and, to a lesser extent, testosterone. BMD in postmenopausal women declines at a higher rate than in men, due perhaps to the more abrupt onset of estrogen reduction. The decline in BMD in men typically lags by at least 5–10 years, depending on their degree of resistance training.

> ***BMD is our best, if imperfect, approximation of fracture risk.***

Proper exercise and nutrition are essential for minimizing osteoporosis. Bone density, muscle strength, and coordination are equally important in preventing fractures. Calcium, vitamin D, vitamin K, vitamin A, and diet acidity can all impact BMD and potentially influence fracture risk.

Calcium absorption

Calcium sources include food (such as dairy, green leafy vegetables and beans) and calcium supplements, although supplements are not ideal sources of calcium, given that heart attacks and prostate cancer have reportedly been associated with calcium supplementation. If supplements are to be used, they should be taken with vitamin D, which is important for absorption. Organic calcium supplements (calcium orotate) have superior bioavailability compared with inorganic supplements (calcium carbonate).

> ***Other conditions that can lead to a less than optimal absorption include reduced stomach acidity (possibly iatrogenic), a high-fiber diet (over 40 g per day), sesame seeds, almonds and oxalate-binding agents found in vegetables such as beets, spinach and rhubarb, if eaten simultaneously with calcium.***

Calcium availability varies from source to source. In spinach, the availability can be as low as 5% of the calcium listed on the package because it bound to oxalate, which makes it much less available. Calcium is critical in the signaling of numerous metabolic pathways. If serum calcium levels are low, the bones' calcium reserves will be used, thereby reducing BMD.

Table 6.1

Calcium Absorbed from Foods

Food	Estimated Calcium Absorption (%)
Milk or yogurt (whole, 2%, 1% and skim)	32.1
Cheddar cheese	32.1
Vegetables	
Bok choy	53.8
Kale	49.3
Chinese spinach	8.4
Broccoli	61
Rhubarb	8.5
Cabbage	52.7
Spinach	5.1
Almonds	21.0
Sesame seeds	21.0

Vitamin D and bone health

Vitamin D is essential for regulating calcium and phosphorus levels, given that it helps absorb calcium. Vitamin D deficiency has been implicated in a broad range of disorders, ranging from osteoporosis to heart disease. Contrary to many popular web pages, vitamin D is very difficult to obtain from the diet. Eggs, halibut, cod, and dover sole are reasonable sources, but sunlight is the simplest way to achieve proper vitamin D levels.

Reduced vitamin D intake and/or production are associated with an increased risk of falls among the elderly. Risks are reduced by 20% with vitamin D supplementation. The risk of hip and vertebral fractures are reduced with the daily intake of 700–800 IU of vitamin D.

If calcium is added to the vitamin D intake, fracture rates are further reduced. A number of authors have recommended sufficient supplementation to meet plasma vitamin D levels of 60–80 ng/ml. Approximately 2000–5000 IU are needed daily to reach such levels, depending on sunlight exposure and starting levels. Vitamin D can be toxic, but rarely at the above listed supplementation level. It is prudent, however, to monitor vitamin D levels until steady states are achieved, accounting for seasonal variation.

Vitamin D supplementation, in the absence of sufficient sunlight exposure, should be performed with vitamin D3.

Table 6.2

Vitamin D Dose

Vitamin D Dose	
Vitamin D deficiency	<20 ng/ml
Vitamin D insufficiency	20–29 ng/ml
Our recommendation	40–70 ng/ml

Vitamin K and bone health

Vegetable sources of vitamin K include green leafy vegetables (e.g., kale, spinach, and mustard greens), leeks, and cruciferous vegetables such as broccoli, cauliflower, and Brussels sprouts. Garnishing or herbs containing substantial vitamin K include capers, parsley, and black peppercorns. Fruit sources include kiwi and blueberries. The daily vitamin K intake recommended by the Institute of Medicine is at least 75 µg , but other sources recommend 120 µg/day for men and 90 µg/day for women.

Vitamin K is important for bone health. The NHS has shown a 30% reduction in hip fractures in women who take at least 110 µg/day of vitamin K, and women who ate 1 serving of green leafy vegetables per day had a 50% reduction in hip fractures compared with those who ate 1 serving per week. The Framingham Heart Study showed data supporting the role of vitamin K in reducing hip fractures in both men and women. Vitamin K1 is the form of vitamin K found in most dietary sources. It is converted into K2 within the body.

Dietary factors that might be counterproductive for BMD include high levels of caffeine (4 or more cups of coffee or soda per day), excess soda consumption, long-term high dietary protein, and excess vitamin A intake. Carbonation, however, is not a risk factor for reduced BMD.

The mechanism behind soda's risk is possibly related to its excess phosphoric acid. Studies have shown increased rates of reduced BMD, even in individuals who drank uncaffeinated colas. Excess phosphoric acid can lead to increased parathyroid hormone secretion, which causes the release of calcium from bone stores to bind with the phosphorous. It is possible that the consumption of phosphorous with calcium sources reduces the bioavailability of dietary calcium by binding it in the small intestine before it can be absorbed. A number of authors contend that the amount of phosphorous in cola is insufficient to have an effect. Due to the lack of information on cola extracts, it is possible that they harbor inherent elements that facilitate reduced BMD.

Long-term high dietary protein (>95 g/day) is potentially linked to increased fracture risk through increased bone resorption of calcium by the stimulation of parathyroid hormone.

Vitamin A and bone health

Excess vitamin A (above 3 mg in one study) leads to a 1.48 relative risk of hip fracture. Current recommended dosages are 900 μg/day for men and 700 μg/day for women. Beta-carotene is the best source of vitamin A, and its intake has not been linked to increased fracture.

The Myth of Alcohol Safety

Alcohol intake

Not needed, but if you are to indulge, try wine.

The risks of alcohol include increased rates of certain malignancies, liver disease, pancreatitis, dementia, stroke, neuropathy, atrial fibrillation, hypertension, cardiomyopathies, and compound psychiatric illnesses such as depression, anxiety, and suicidal tendencies.

The benefits of alcohol, when use is moderate, include an improved heart disease risk profile and reduced mortality. Bearing in mind that similar gains in the heart disease risk profile can be achieved with nutrition and exercise modification, there is no unique benefit to alcohol use.

According to the American Heart Association (AHA), the recommended level of alcohol consumption is an average of 1–2 drinks per day for men and 1 for women. A drink is defined as 1 oz or 14 g of 100-proof spirits. This approximates to a 5% 12-oz (355 ml) beer, a 12% 5-oz (148 ml) glass of wine and 1.5 oz (44 ml) of 40-proof spirits. The AHA recommendations are considered moderate alcohol intake. Heavy alcohol intake is up to 3.5 drinks per day for men and up to 2.5 drinks per day for women. Very heavy alcohol intake is above these limits. Heavy and very heavy drinking, by almost all definitions, is alcoholism and needs to be addressed as such for treatment.

The AHA cautions those who do not drink against beginning to drink. The implication, despite acclaimed health benefits, is that drinking is not necessary for healthy living and carries certain risks.

Figure 6.1

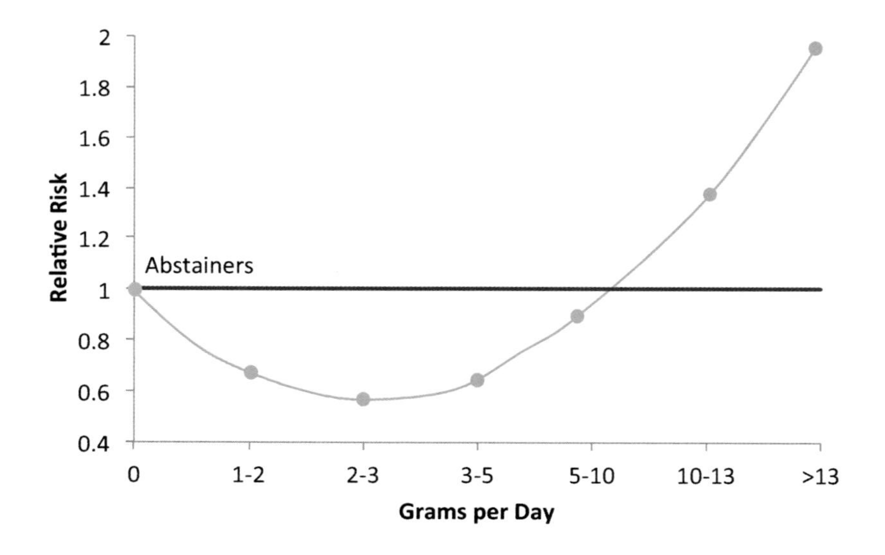

Heart disease

A population study that assessed the risk of heart disease in over 4000 patients showed that moderate alcohol consumption lowered known heart disease markers (HDL in particular), whereas high and very high-volume drinkers had high blood pressure, neutralizing the beneficial effects of increased HDL. A moderate drinker was classified as one who consumed 1–13 drinks per week. A high-volume or very high-volume drinker was defined as one who consumed 14–34 drinks/week and >35 drinks/week, respectively. The systolic and diastolic blood pressures of the high-volume drinkers were increased by approximately 5 mm Hg and 3 mm Hg, respectively. The overall risk of heart disease rose from 4.31% to 4.90% in a 10-year period. The relationship between alcohol and known heart disease risks is therefore J-shaped.

There is an initial drop in risk with moderate drinking, but the risk then rises with progressively greater drinking.

Interestingly, wine consumption had the most substantial increases in HDL levels, whereas beer and spirits increased TG levels. Alcohol is a toxin, and, as with many toxins, the body might be able to manage a small amount for a limited period. Similarly, too much alcohol can overtax the body's ability to detoxify. Heart disease is currently the single greatest cause of mortality; however, the major disease directly and indirectly resulting from alcohol consumption is cancer. When heart disease is effectively reduced by proper nutrition and exercise, cancer will likely be the leading cause of death. Cancer, however, involves a much more heterogeneous group of diseases (and causes) than heart disease. Tackling cancer will therefore require a longer and more complex strategy, one that will undoubtedly involve proper nutrition and exercise practices, given that numerous cancers are avoidable through lifestyle changes.

Reducing alcohol consumption reduces your risk of cancer.

Figure 6.2

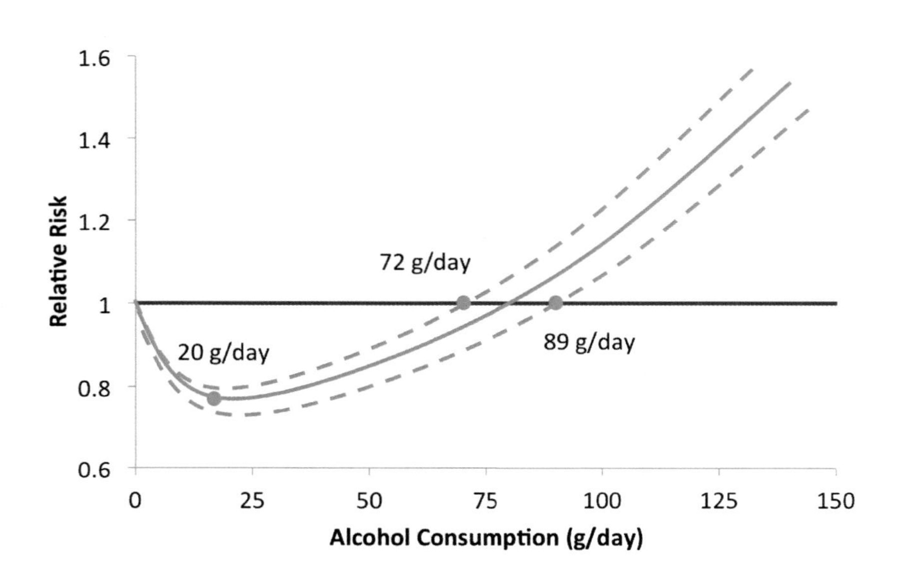

Cancer

Especially with spirits

In 1988, the International Agency for Research on Cancer declared alcohol a carcinogen. In 2014, the World Cancer Report directly refuted the "responsible drinking" theme and formally stated no amount of alcohol is safe when considering cancer risk.

Increasing evidence suggests not only a modest risk of increased heart disease with heavy alcohol intake but a potential increase in the risk of cancer. A population study performed in European countries with over 350,000 men and women aged 37–70 showed 10% of cancers in men and 3% of cancers in women were associated with heavy alcohol intake (more than 2 drinks per day for men and more than 1 drink per day for women).

Malignancies causally linked to alcohol use include oropharyngeal, laryngeal, esophageal, colorectal, hepatic, breast (female) and potentially pancreatic tumors. There is epidemiological data that suggest a strong association, rather than causation, between alcohol use and leukemia, multiple myeloma, and cervical, vulvar, vaginal, and skin cancers. There is conflicting evidence for bladder, lung, and stomach cancers. The total number of deaths we can therefore potentially link at this time to alcohol use is more than 21,284, which is >3.7% of US cancer deaths as of 2009.

Self-reporting methods used for collecting data for epidemiological studies can underestimate the number of deaths and the strength of the association between alcohol use and cancers.

Causal mechanisms of alcohol use and cancer are still being investigated. Direct carcinogens found in alcohol include acetaldehyde, acrylamide, aflatoxins, arsenic, benzene, cadmium, ethanol (the most prevalent), ethyl carbamate, formaldehyde, and lead.

Breast cancer in women is often hormone-sensitive, such that increased estrogen levels that can accompany chronic alcohol use might increase the probability of malignancy in certain patients.

Smoking and alcohol use often coexist in the social setting. Ironically, the carcinogens from cigarettes might be more readily absorbed because ethanol acts as a solvent, putting the oropharyngeal system at particular risk. This increased risk is strongly supported in the literature, to the extent that avoiding cigarettes and alcohol is estimated to be capable of preventing 80% of oral cancer cases and 90% of laryngeal cancer cases.

Spirits (distilled alcohol, often 40 proof or higher) are linked to esophageal cancer.

Does the type of alcohol matter?

- *Wine is probably the healthiest type of alcohol, but most of the benefits of alcohol can be achieved through other lifestyle changes.*

Data suggest that the type of alcohol does affect the risk of alcohol consumption. In short, wine consumption is probably the safest type, followed by beer and closely by spirits. Cancer risk is the most substantial difference among the various forms of alcohol, with spirits showing the highest cancer risk and wine the lowest.

Figure 6.3

Mortality and the Consumption of Various Types of Alcohol

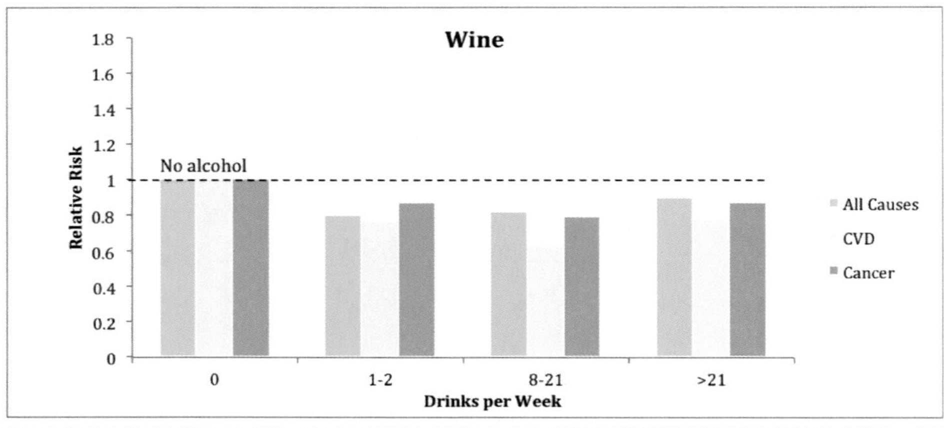

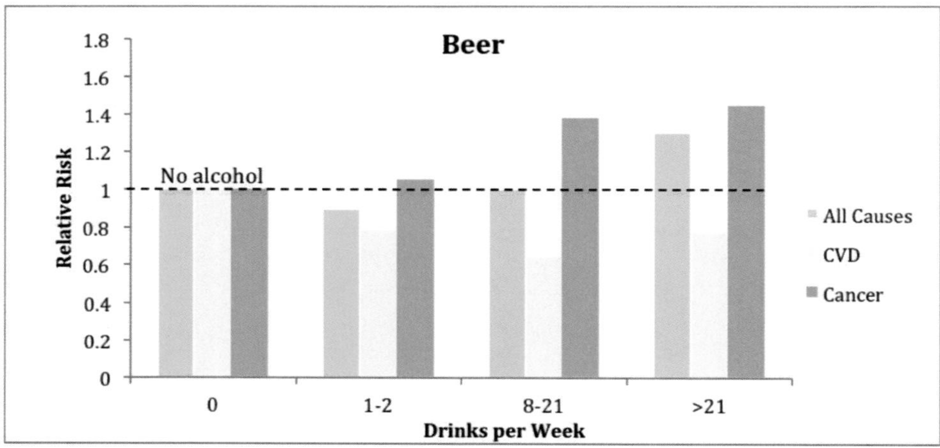

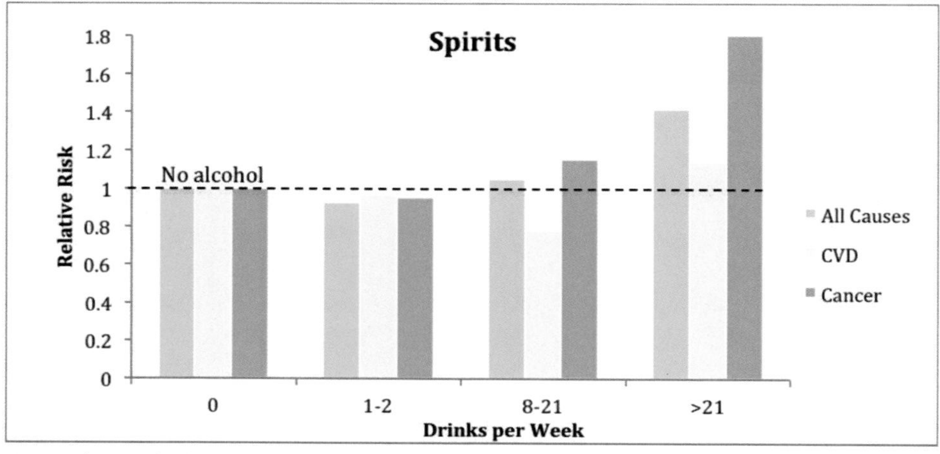

CVD: cardiovascular disease

**This is one of very few studies that distinguishes the effects of different types of alcohol.*

Cognition

When the various sources of alcohol are considered, the data suggest that wine is more protective than spirits or beer. The risks for all forms of dementia have been reported as lower with mild to moderate alcohol consumption. Risk reduction could be as much as 25%–35%, with most benefits reported in wine drinkers.

Worse cognition and dementia have been reported in heavy drinkers (5–6 drinks per day) and in individuals with the APOEε4 allele.

Sleep and alcohol use

They don't mix

Sleep quality usually declines as we age, and the use of alcohol adds to the challenge of getting restful sleep. Although alcohol can induce sleep, the sleep is characterized by a initial sleep cycle that is associated with a shorter REM sleep stage and a longer non-REM sleep stage (short wave sleep). This consolidated effect is dose-related. Withdrawal symptoms then occur, resulting in shallow sleep, multiple awakenings, REM rebound-associated nightmares, sweating, and increased brain activation. Reduced total REM sleep is most prominently shown by moderate to high doses of alcohol.

Alcohol suppresses plasma GH by 75% at night (0.8g/kg), the equivalent of approximately four 14-g drinks. All measures of GH are affected by alcohol. GH returns to normal levels on nights when alcohol is not consumed, even after chronic use. Less alcohol results in less GH suppression; however, because GH is so important in the mechanisms of recovery and repair, alcohol's interference can take a substantial toll.

Inflammation from alcohol intake

Both pro-inflammatory and anti-inflammatory changes can occur

Changes in the inflammatory response associated with alcohol intake are shown in both the acute and chronic state, each exhibiting different responses. Both states are modulated, at least in part, through monocytes (derived from bone marrow). Gram-negative bacteria in the gastrointestinal tract secrete endotoxins in response to alcohol.

With acute alcohol intake, there is an impaired binding of NFκB and transactivation, reducing the production of anti-inflammatory TNFα. Chronic alcohol intake is associated with increased TNFα and a net pro-inflammatory state.

In the elderly, light alcohol intake is associated with lower IL-6 and C-reactive protein levels.

Summary: Alcohol Intake

Although alcohol can have mild cardiovascular benefits with light to moderate drinking, it is our experience that light to moderate drinking is often interspersed with episodic binge-type drinking and/or smoking and other indulgences, including increased intake of less than optimal food.

> ***If you want to indulge in drinking even 1–2 glasses of a wine per day, it should be with the understanding that you are making an allowance for a toxin, rather than doing it under the guise of health promotion.***

We emphasize that there is probably more of a linear relationship between alcohol use and the overall impact on health, rather than a U-shaped or threshold-based relationship. Therefore, light alcohol use is associated with a slight increased risk, rather than it being healthy up to a point. In a patient who also does not sleep well, has obesity and does not exercise, this small risk can be significant.

Alcohol imparts heart disease benefits, to a limited degree. In populations with low heart disease incidence, studies have shown no improvement in mortality in those who drink mildly to moderately compared with those who do not drink. Given that the benefits of heart disease can be achieved with other lifestyle changes, it is arguable that alcohol is not cumulatively beneficial to survival but rather one of several ways to reduce heart disease. Given that there is a clear connection between alcohol ingestion and cancer risk, we believe in advising patients to strive for zero alcohol consumption, especially when they are consistently involved in lifestyles that reduce heart disease. All things considered, we advise our patients to minimize or eliminate alcohol consumption.

For those who wish to continue to consume alcohol, we suggest the following:

1. Less is best: Lower alcohol consumption adds to improved health and longevity. Wine is probably the safest choice.
2. As with calories and carbohydrates, be aware of how much you consume.
3. Limit consumption to 1.5 drinks daily for men and 1 drink daily for women.
4. Take a holiday from drinking now and then. It helps the liver recover.
5. The caloric intake (non-alcoholic) during drinking days can be several hundred calories higher than during nondrinking days. Weight management goals can therefore be significantly impaired.

We ask patients for a direct quantification of alcohol intake per day and week, including the type and social setting. We assume this represents a *minimum* level consumed.

Green Tea

Drink it up; 3-4 cups a day. Learn how to make it properly so you can enjoy it.

There are 20 mg of caffeine per 100-ml cup of green tea prepared at 90°C (194°F), with 10 g of tea leaf steeped in 430 ml of water for 1 minute. By comparison, coffee contains approximately 60 mg of caffeine per 100 ml, or thrice the amount contained in green tea. Steeping is an art in itself, with some teas requiring shorter steeping times and cooler water temperatures than others. Most tea steeping occurs in 2–4 minutes at temperatures lower than 85°C (185°F). The key health factors of green tea (unoxidized) include the following:

◊ Polyphenols (epigallocatechin gallate [EGCG])

- Flavonoids (anti-oxidant, anti-carcinogenic)
- Catechins (EGCG)

- Theaflavins (particularly black tea)
- Tannins (which increase with steeping time)

Green tea is probably one of the most valuable dietary additions we can recommend to patients (in addition to omega-3 fatty acids). Extracts are healthy supplements, and green tea is rich in polyphenols, such as EGCG, which has thermogenic effects and promotes fat oxidization. Studies have shown that EGCG is significant in promoting fat loss (especially visceral) and restores insulin sensitivity. Similar effects have been described with high-protein diets. Green tea extract has been shown to increase fat oxidation by 17% and glucose sensitivity by 14%. Green tea is also rich in L-theanine, which is well known for its capacity for stress relief, mood balance, immune function, and premenstrual symptom relief.

Green tea with a concomitant exercise program further promotes fat oxidation in both the liver and muscle. Exercise endurance is also higher in animals administered green tea extract.

Theanine is found in abundance in green tea, accounting for 50% of its amino acid properties. It increases alpha waves and decreases beta waves and is considered a relaxant rather than an agent that causes drowsiness. Theanine reduces heart rate and blood pressure, reversing the effects of similar doses of caffeine. Results from experimental studies indicate that when L-theanine (250 mg) is taken in conjunction with the caffeine in green tea (150 mg), alertness is improved and fatigue is reduced. In the brain, L-theanine reduces oxidative stress and inhibits neuronal cell death. As little as 30 mg of theanine has been reported to improve mood and cognition, with a significant increase in α-wave activity. In patients with premenstrual symptoms, 200 mg/day of L-theanine helped stabilize mood and reduced irritability, crying and other symptoms. Green tea and theanine have been shown to improve T-cell function and reduce cold and flu symptoms. Other healthful ingredients in green tea are shown in the table below.

Theanine Dose: 50-200 mg/day PO

Table 6.3

Healthful Ingredients in Green Tea

Ingredients	Benefit
Vitamin C	Anti-infection and anti-cancer
Caffeine and L-theanine	Cognitive
EGCG Beta Carotene	Anti-cancer
Catechins	Anti-infection Increases fat burning (lipolysis) Lowers cholesterol lipoproteins (LDL) Protects neurons; may reduce Alzheimers Reduces halitosis **Reduces visceral fat** **Reduces DMII** **Reduces heart disease** Reduces Mortality in Women and Men

EGCG: epigallocatechin gallate; LDL: low-density lipoproteins

**Per standard cup*

Taken from http://authoritynutrition.com/top-10-evidence-based-health-benefits-of-green-tea/

There are few human studies that have directly assessed the effects of green tea on cognition and mental status. One study in a Japanese population convincingly showed improved mental status, based on the results of the Mini Mental State Examination (MMSE). Given the fact that Alzheimer's disease is consistently preceded by cognitive decline, the improved MMSE scores begin to quantify how much green tea can reduce the risk of dementia, although the study did not directly study dementia as a diagnosis. Interestingly, the study suggests that caffeine is *not* the active ingredient in improved cognitive function by comparing the results of coffee drinkers who ingested 3 times more caffeine on average than the tea drinkers. The coffee drinkers did not show nearly the degree of protection in cognitive function as the green tea drinkers, despite having more caffeine. In fact, coffee was found to be a risk for cognitive decline, although it was not statistically significant.

Figure 6.4

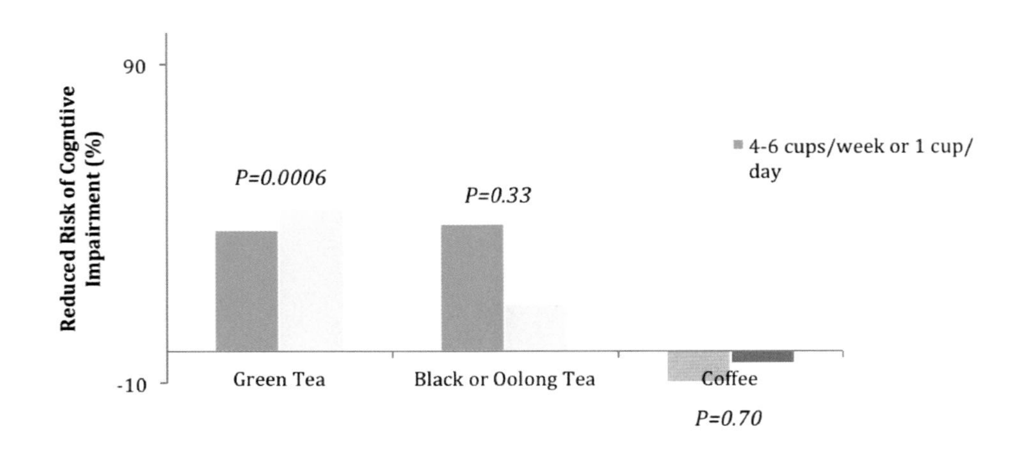

The results of the study showed that green tea consumption and improved MMSE scores were dose-related, further supporting the validity of the study. Those individuals who drank at least 2 cups of tea per day compared with those who drank approximately 1 cup per day showed progressively better MMSE scores.

Neuroimaging studies have shown that green tea extract modulates the activity in the dorsal lateral prefrontal cortex, which is known to mediate working memory, an ability commonly affected by age-related cognitive decline. Thus, the neuroimaging studies support the neuroprotective effect on dementia of green tea through a plausible mechanism.

Nutraceuticals

Get your core nutrition established before becoming distracted by nutraceuticals

Nutraceuticals are natural compounds reported to enhance natural functions. Chinese and Ayurvedic medicine have employed forms of nutraceuticals for centuries. A number of nutraceuticals are found naturally in the human body, such as amino acids, cofactors, vitamins, and minerals. Nutraceuticals and supplements are generally not considered "drugs" in the way pharmaceuticals are.

The literature is inconclusive as to the safety and efficacy of any given nutraceutical. Studies on nutraceuticals are rare, small, short in length, often not experimental, and frequently do not have control groups even when they are experimental.

The "problem of proof" is rooted in the polyvalent nature of nutrition, more so than with other areas of study such as exercise and hormone replacement therapy. Unlike drugs, nutrients work in complex networks modulated by homeostatic mechanisms, with effects that can require years to manifest. Randomized controlled studies are nearly impossible due to the complexity of nutrition among the various participants. Alternate study designs are required, but without a series of global indices for each nutrient, the task of proving the effectiveness of individual nutraceuticals and micronutrients (vitamins and minerals) is daunting.

Nutraceuticals are subject to much laxer regulation than pharmaceuticals. The consumer is therefore burdened with a number of issues such as the purity and potency of nutraceuticals, which are often entirely the consumer's responsibility to research. Toxicity is a real possibility. Drug interactions are often overlooked, and if patients do not report their nutraceuticals in the list of medications they are taking, drug interactions become more likely. As with food, the quality of the source of the product is critical. Consumer laboratories review numerous nutraceuticals for the validity of their claims, purity and toxic/contamination elements, such as lead.

Alpha-lipoic acid (ALA) has a broad range of benefits. ALA increases the production of glutathione, which is an antioxidant that reduces the buildup of proteins in the eyes that can lead to blurry vision. ALA has also been shown to protect the optic nerve and stabilize intraocular pressure.

ALA improves insulin sensitivity in overweight adults and reduces related symptoms such as pain, numbness, tingling and burning sensations.

Dosage: 75-600 mg/day

Turmeric (Curcuma Longa) has significant anti-inflammatory properties, and its active constituent is curcumin. On a molecular level, turmeric has been shown to modulate inflammation through NFκB, TNF, COX-2, IL-2 and IL-6. Turmeric has been used in traditional medicine for liver ailments. Although turmeric shows poor bioavailability, new clinical trials with phospholipid complexes of curcumin have provided a better delivery system.

Milk thistle contains silymarin, a bioflavonoid comprised of silybin, silydianin, and silychristin. These agents act to bind the outer cell membrane of hepatocytes, preventing harmful toxins from entering. Silymarin enhances glutathione and superoxide dismutase and stimulates regeneration in damaged liver cells.

Dosage: 250 mg PO QD

Magnesium orotate is an essential mineral for calcium and potassium integration, nerve and muscle impulses, enzymatic reactions, heart and muscle health, glucose homeostasis, and a variety of other critical cellular functions.

Magnesium orotate is used to treat symptoms of magnesium deficiency, including diabetes, hypertension, dementia, osteoporosis, migraines, asthma, myocardial infarctions, arrhythmias, and atherosclerosis. The compound can improve flow-mediated dilation by 12% after 6 months with 730 mg/day. In patients with diabetes, magnesium orotate has been shown to improve insulin sensitivity and glycemic control. Athletes use magnesium orotate to increase endurance. The benefits of magnesium orotate over other magnesium supplements include its higher intracellular and mitochondrial concentration.

Dosage: 500–1000 mg/day

L-arginine is an amino acid and a substrate for nitric oxide synthase. The acid has been shown to promote vasodilation and reduce systolic blood pressure by 5–6 mm Hg and diastolic blood pressure by 2–3 mm Hg. Long-term treatment with approximately 8 g/day has been shown to improve insulin sensitivity and glucose metabolism, especially in concomitant athletic training. The acid also improves endothelial function and reduces oxidative stress and adipokinin release in patients with DMII.

Dosage: 8.3 g/day

Sweetened beverages

Naturally and artificially sweetened beverages have significant metabolic implications both for patients who have obesity and those who don't. Fructose-sweetened beverages in populations without obesity increase postprandial TG levels. The 24-hour insulin secretion is reduced, and leptin levels are lowered, compared with the effects of glucose-sweetened beverages.

Fructose-sweetened beverages consumed by patients with obesity produced similar results as those demonstrated in patients without obesity: increased postprandial TG levels, reduced insulin secretion, and blunted diurnal leptin response. In patients with obesity and insulin resistance, postprandial TG levels were further increased, which suggests that fructose can exacerbate an already adverse metabolic profile in patients with obesity.

> ***A diet high in added sugars is associated with increased markers of heart disease.***

An analysis of data gathered for the cross-sectional population study of the National Health and Nutrition Examination Survey (NHANES) showed a linear inverse relationship between HDL and simple sugar intake. HDL levels ranged from 58.7 mg/dl in participants who consumed the 5% recommended limit (or less) of added sugars to 47.7 mg/dl in participants who consumed 25% of their total intake in the form of added sugar. HDL levels of 40 mg/dl for men and 50 mg/dl for women are considered a risk factor for heart disease. TG levels were directly related to increased sugar consumption, ranging from 105 mg/dl to 123 mg/dl.

In randomized controlled studies, participants with obesity and those with normal weight who consumed sugar-sweetened (glucose, fructose, sucrose) beverages had increased markers of heart disease, including high-sesnsitivity C-reactive protein (which increased by 60%–109%) and fasting glucose (which increased by 4%–9%), from all sugar types. A higher proportion of LDL (more atherosclerotic) was shown with increased fructose intake. Increased leptin levels were shown with glucose intake only. These results occurred in as little as 3 weeks. Thus, higher glucose and fructose consumption creates an impaired glucose metabolism, a more plaque-promoting cholesterol profile and a proinflammatory state in patients with and without obesity.

Fruit and fructose: Impact on glycemic index

A 6-month, parallel controlled study of patients with diabetes showed that, in conjunction with a low-GI diet (controlled for fiber), low-GI fruit and high-fiber bread consumption was associated with lower HbA1c levels, lower systolic blood pressure (4%), and lower heart disease risk (increased HDL by up to 7.3%), while maintaining a stable BMI. Although fruits range from 50 to 103 GI units, the temperate fruits tend to be on the lower end, at less than 70 GI units. These types of fruits include apples, pears, citrus fruits, berries, nectarines, peaches, and plums. Tropical fruits tend have >70 GI units and include fruits such as bananas, mangos, guavas, grapes, watermelon, and cantaloupe. In the study, fruit consumption at baseline was approximately 1.4 servings per day, half of which was low GI fruit. By the end of the 6-month period, the low-GI fruit consumption had doubled in the low-GI fruit diet group.

Up to 3 servings per day of low-GI fruit was associated with the most substantial reduction in heart disease risk.

Specifically, citrus and berries were more closely associated with reduced HbA1c. Apple consumption was negatively correlated with TG levels, total cholesterol/HDL levels, and heart disease risk, and was positively associated with HDL levels. Berry intake was negatively correlated with blood pressure and fasting blood glucose. Berry intake was positively correlated with TG levels.

Studies have shown that small increases in fructose intake (7–10 g) can serve as a catalyst in priming glucose metabolism. The result of the priming is shown in MRI spectroscopy studies in which there is a reduction of postprandial glucose concentrations with increased liver glycogen synthesis (as an alternative to fatty acid synthesis and TG storage). In patients with diabetes, a low-dose infusion of fructose restores the inhibitory effect of hyperglycemia, which reduces hepatic glucose output. The molecular mechanism is thought to act through an increase in fructose-1-phosphate levels, displacing glucokinase from the bound position in the nucleus, allowing it to be effectively translocated to the cell surface, where it fulfills its function of facilitating glucose uptake into the hepatocyte.

> ***Large amounts of fructose (17%–25% of dietary energy), which is commonly incorporated into many food and drink products, results in unfavorable glucose metabolism and consequently unfavorable cholesterol profiles.***

This type of dietary intake results in high fasting and postprandial TG levels, higher LDL levels, higher visceral fat body composition, and impaired carbohydrate tolerance. These changes are known to increase the risk of DMII and heart disease.

The parallel study described above focused on fruit and high-fiber bread in replacing high GI diet content with low GI diet content. The authors continue to support the low GI food plan as beneficial in minimizing the risk of DMII and heart disease. The authors state that up to 3 servings of fruit a day can be associated with a reduced risk of DMII and heart disease. Given that both low GI fruit and high-fiber bread diet modifications result in independent but similar trends of reduced DMII and heart disease, it is not necessarily the fruit or the high-fiber bread but the reduced GI factor that is the most significant factor in risk reduction. However, of the two products, the one more likely to have added nutrient value is fruit. Fruits arguably have a similar or higher quality of fiber than that found in bread products. Fruit also contains minerals, antioxidants, and phenols that have been associated (though not clearly established as causative) with reduced oxidative stress, reduced systolic blood pressure, improved glucose control, and overall improved heart disease-related outcomes.

Summary: Fruit and Fructose

We recommend 2–3 servings of low GI fruit per day for patients with and without diabetes. Patients with diabetes are encouraged to eat naturally occurring sugars but to not go beyond 10% of their diet. We suggest 1–2 low GI fruits. The goal is to replace less healthy carbohydrate sources with healthier ones.

NutraSweet® and other artificial sweeteners (aspartame)

Artificial sweeteners are consumed in massive amounts. Many of these consumers are patients with diabetes or high BMI who are struggling with caloric and blood glucose control. Aspartame, AceK, saccharin, and sucralose are common manufactured intense sweeteners. Aspartame and AceK are similarly sweet, approximately 200 times sweeter than sucrose. Saccharin is approximately 300 times as sweet as sucrose, and sucralose is approximately 600 times as sweet as sucrose. Less commonly used sweeteners include cyclamate, additives such as alcohols, neotame, stevia, erythritol, xylitol, and tagatose. The use of such high-intensity sweeteners naturally raises the question of their impact on gastrointestinal signaling in appetite regulation. Do they have similar or overlapping effects as glucose or other naturally occurring simple sugars?

In nematodes, aspartame has been associated with a reduction of intestinal fat deposit. AceK was associated with increased intestinal fat deposit in the presence of insulin resistance. In a small controlled study in humans, AceK was associated with marginal increases in the blood glucose response, whereas aspartame and saccharin were not. None had effects on satiation. There was an initial concern of an increased rate of brain tumors, lymphoma, and leukemia; however, studies have not demonstrated a correlation between aspartame and increased cancer rates.

We recommend against artificial substances of any type in food products from a common sense standpoint and because of the increased costs of processing, the reduced nutrient value, and the studies that suggest their negative health consequences. Artificial sweeteners facilitate an unhealthy relationship with food products, promoting a preference for excess sugary tastes.

Salt

It is overly managed. Stay away from processed foods and you'll be fine.

Unless a patient has hypertension, we suggest that salt be used freely, according to an individual's desire for more or less salt. When processed foods are eliminated or nearly eliminated, consuming excess sodium becomes less of a problem. If processed foods are still part of the diet, therapy and support should be focused on removing them before worrying about salt monitoring.

> ***The AHA sodium recommendation of <1.5 g/day was as misguided as the recommendation in past decades for following a low-fat diet.***

These recommendations lead to untenable adherence. The Dietary Guidelines for Americans recommended an intake of 2.3 g of salt per day in people younger than 50, and 1.5 g/day for those 50 and older. These recommendations are currently undergoing changes.

If you consume less than 3 g of sodium per day, you have a 25% increased morbidity and mortality risk compared with those who consume 4–6 g of daily sodium. However, sodium consumption in excess of 7 g per day can place you at a 15% increased risk of morbidity and mortality compared with those in the 4–6 g/day range.

Thus, if a range needs to be provided, 4–6 g per day is a sound recommendation. For patients with mild hypertension, we recommend the low end of the 4–6 g/day range, followed by serial home-monitored blood pressure readings several times a day over a 2-week period. When a normal blood pressure pattern is established, we suggest a deliberate 1g/day additional intake for 2 weeks with continued blood pressure monitoring to assess the changes. If there is no change, you can continue the process to establish that increased salt intake does not increase your blood pressure.

Email us your questions! We would love to answer them.

There are many more topics of interest, and although we would like to cover them all, time and space do not permit. Please visit *BeneVitaHealth.com* and send us a topic you would like us to address.

Conclusion

Part VIII

A critical concept you should be familiar with by now is that fat is an inflammatory organ. It secretes several hormones and pro-inflammatory agents. Visceral fat is pro-inflammatory and is strongly implicated in premature heart disease due to these traits.

In contrast, muscle is an anti-inflammatory organ.

Inflammation imbalance is strongly implicated in the leading causes of death, namely heart disease and cancer, and in the conditions that precede them. Inflammation affects a wide range of other diseases and, together with obesity and hormone (insulin, leptin, and incretin) resistance, is a precursor of metabolic syndrome.

Both inflammation and insulin resistance have direct and indirect roles in metabolic syndrome, the constellation of disorders that precede the formal diagnosis of DMII and heart disease.

Metabolic syndrome is useful as a concept to describe an intermediary state of one or more clinical conditions that precede the formal diagnosis of DMII, which, in turn, is strongly implicated in many cases of premature heart disease. The syndrome is comprised of obesity, a trend toward insulin resistance, hypertension, and poor cholesterol levels (dyslipidemia), all of which are consequences of excess adiposity.

Leptin plays a major role in appetite regulation, as do incretins and insulin. Inflammation and hormone insensitivity therefore play major roles in dysregulated appetites.

We prefer a low-carb approach for everyone; however, given that cardiometabolic health improves with visceral fat loss, the only thing that matters is what you can maintain. Pushing an ideal that you cannot keep is not useful to you. What matters most is body fat reduction, not the particular food plan. All studies considered, it is apparent that they *all* can work, if executed with *high compliance.* The compliance rates for groups as a whole are higher with the Zone and Mediterranean diets and lower with the Atkins and Ornish diets. Weight Watchers might be appealing for others.

All healthy diets exclude sugar, flour (any variation), and corn. However, most of us cannot begin by making such drastic changes all at once. We therefore advise you on the ideal scenario, planting a seed but without trying to force it so early in your transformation. It is perhaps as instructive to us as clinicians as it is to you to view various dietary interventions (such as low-carb or moderate-protein diets) as tools that may be used either alone or in combination to manipulate the physiological systems to achieve an improved clinical state. In terms of diets, we should view people as individuals and not as countries, eras of human evolution or members of macronutrient camps. People have individual genomics, hedonics, compensatory behaviors and physiologies. "Compliance is king", and high compliance underpins any successful nutritional or exercise intervention. The nutritional prescription, as with every prescription a physician writes, is an individual one based upon your individual needs analysis.

You are faced with several health choices every day, mainly, what to eat and whether to exercise. The choices lie along a spectrum from poor to ideal. For you to progress, you simply have to shift the weighted average of those decisions toward ideal. Make more frequent ideal choices. Perfect is the enemy of good, and striving for perfect choices all the time will result in failure. Failure leads to frustration, and frustration leads to abandoning the project. Progress is made by simply doing things a little better than you did yesterday. Each day the goal should be the same and should be independent of the previous day's success or failure. In this way, our good health is not a destination to arrive at but a journey we are always on. Our good health is something that cannot be provided to us but rather something we earn.

Although heart disease is the leading cause of mortality, it will slowly begin to decline. Cancer is the second leading cause of death in the US, with mortality rates very close to those of heart disease, and is a much more heterogeneous group of diseases. Cancer will likely become the next focus for reducing mortality, as heart disease is eventually controlled through improved nutrition and exercise.

We hope this chapter has given you food for thought. The amount of information about nutrition can be daunting. Even more daunting is the apparently conflicting information that is so often published. This is unlikely to change soon due to the nature of nutrition and the inability to create truly controlled trials.

Nevertheless, you have the essence of what you need to aim for. When you are ready, pick a program that makes sense to you, one that you think you can adhere to for 4 weeks. Then strive to find a balance, one that you can live with indefinitely. Strive simply to make better nutritional choices with the new information you have from this chapter and the insights you gain from your 4-week effort. Keep experimenting with what works for you. Find your sweet spot in the figure below.

Figure 8.1

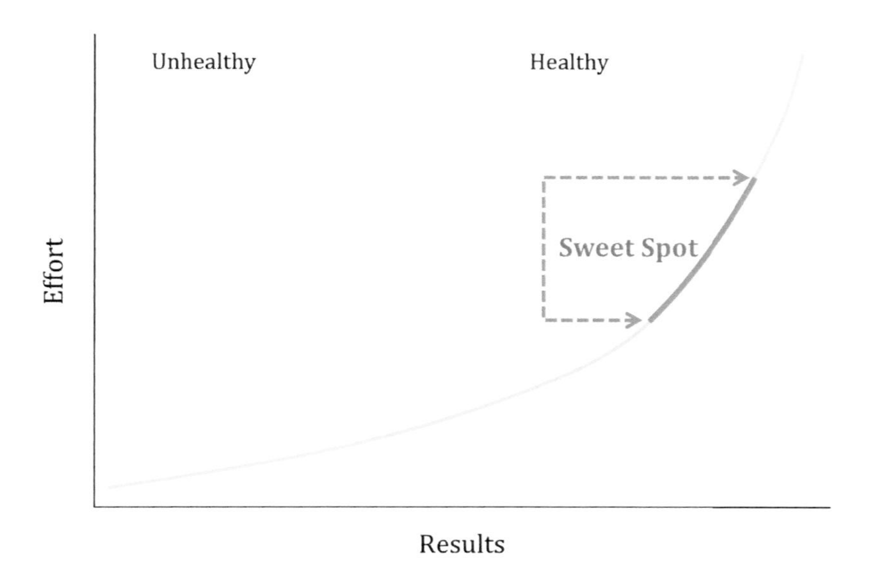

A note on conceptual models

In medicine, as with all science, we develop models that seem to fit based on the available evidence. However, it is common that models need altering. Sometimes, a simple refining of the current model can provide it with more accuracy and utility. Other times, the model has to be discarded and a new one designed. Recognizing when models are wrong or at least in need of refinement is essential for not misguiding the people we care for in medicine. Frankly, the "bad fat" model was wrong and took too long to fix.

A note on the news

All of us, including patients, scientists, nutritionists and clinicians, are constantly bombarded with mixed messages about what is healthy for us and what is not. There are a few reasons for the confusion. The first is the general limitation of observational population-based studies, especially in nutrition. The second is the insurmountable obstacle that the food industry faces, which is to add nutritional value to food and still make a profit. Instead, they have made food abnormally tasty at the expense of nutrition. The third is the media's inherent need to create controversy. This has unfortunately resulted in women losing a decade of the benefits of hormone replacement therapy (including reduced osteoporosis, heart disease and mortality). The comforting truth is that there is nothing glamorous about fresh natural whole foods, and there is not much to add to improve it.

The first challenge for nutritional literature is that we rely heavily on epidemiological data, which is observational data collected from large populations, to determine what is good or healthy for an individual. Therefore, much of what we know about nutrition is that which is *associated* with good health. However, association does not mean causation, which is a critical distinction in deciding what to incorporate into your personal nutritional program. For example, we know healthy people tend to have high vitamin D levels. However, that does not mean that taking vitamin D will create good health in a person with an otherwise unhealthy lifestyle.

In contrast to observational studies, randomized controlled studies (experimental) try to establish cause, rather than association, by keeping all things equal except for the factor being studied. For example, in a theoretical, randomized controlled study determining the effects of vitamin D on health, we would ideally study a group of identical twins in the same climate with the same exact food intake, eating at the same time each day, sleeping the same amount each night, with the same amount of sun exposure each day and the same exercise routine. One of the twins would take vitamin D each day, and the other would not. The time period for the study would be at least 1-10 years. All factors, except for vitamin D, would therefore be controlled. We would than determine what endpoint we would measure to determine the effect on health. Perhaps that endpoint would be how long the twins lived; however, the study would then have to last decades. Another option might be to assess more than one factor, such as inflammation levels and endothelial health, to establish which twin was healthier at the end of the study.

Whatever the measurement or end point, it would have to be established as a validated method of measuring good health. Even that can be challenging. We often associate high LDL levels with poor health because lipids, when exposed to unhealthy blood vessels, tend to create plaques that cause heart attacks and strokes. However, patients with otherwise healthy blood vessels can have high LDL levels and not experience heart attacks. This is why most people who experience heart attacks actually have normal lipid levels. Thus, is measuring lipid levels really a measure of good health? It can be of value but only to a point. High lipids do not cause heart attacks. Any amount of lipids in unhealthy blood vessels can contribute to heart attacks.

Creating randomized controlled trials to prove that X causes Y or that vitamin D intake increases health is nearly impossible. With exercise, it is somewhat easier to control for the most influential elements, such as technique, weight, repetitions and intensity. The science of exercise is therefore more conclusive but still far from definitive. Nutrition is a very challenging topic because of the range of possible influencing factors that are difficult to monitor.

Another reason the nutritional messages are confusing is the result of the competitive food market. In general, competition in most circles breeds excellence. It forces companies to create better products that create greater demand than that of the competitors' products. In the food industry, better products unfortunately do not equate with healthy products. The food industry has created products with prettier pictures on the boxes and catchier punch lines, but these food products are developed for taste, not nutrition. In fact, it is hard to top the nutritional value of fresh natural whole foods. For the past decades, the food industry has given consumers what it could, an empty promise of "better food." Their version of better food is food that is visually appealing and very tasty, what we call highly palatable food. In fact, food is *too palatable,* not naturally palatable. Much of the increased palatability has been achieved by dumping all types of sugar into the food. The high density of sugar leads to calorie-packed foods that lack fiber. Not only has the food become highly palatable, but in the process the food has been robbed of nutrition. Unbeknownst to the consumer, the food has become nutritionally poor. The food industry has thus created highly palatable, energy-dense, nutritionally poor food.

When the consumer demands nutritionally rich foods, the food industry will have no choice in providing these foods. Consumers beware—the food industry will do its utmost to pretend to offer healthy food. They will replace trans fats with unesterified fats, sugar with maltose or cane sugar, real fiber with unidimensional fiber or healthy whole protein with limited proteins. When the food industry begins to offer healthy food, it will look a lot like a farmer's market and nothing else. The profit in such a market is limited to whatever benefit the food industry can provide in terms of distribution. In truth, it is hard to add nutritional value to fresh natural whole foods.

Finally, the media and those who use the media are at fault for drumming up controversy in order to have sell or propagate an agenda. The 2002 WHI trial study results purportedly contradicted decades of clinical experience and literature data that said HRT for women was safe. The NIH and the study group intentionally released misleading headline news that HRT was not safe for women and dramatically and prematurely ended the trial. The 2002 data, when analyzed properly, clearly showed that HRT was safe for women who have no established heart disease. The scientists, however, did not present that data. They presented data that included women who were already at risk (elderly and with established heart disease). Although the trial ended in 2002, the data continued to be collected over the next decade. Each year, more and more data confirmed that HRT for women was safe when started during a specific window. However, the media was accustomed to dissuading clinicians from prescribing HRT and women from demanding it.

It is impractical for the reader to analyze all new literature that emerges. The first thing we suggest is to not react to headlines or Internet hype. Develop a core set of nutritional values today that are well established in the literature and require a high bar before reconsidering them. They will serve you well your entire life. Getting lost in the forest of information is not uncommon. Keep the big picture on nutrition, and the rest becomes points of interest, curiosities, and perhaps food for thought in your personal experiences during your journey. This text will help you establish that core set of values, which we offer you based on our practice's years of analyzing research and professional success in the clinical setting.

Ten Top Tips for finding your nutrition sweet spot

1. Eat whole foods.
2. Obesity is the result of eating too much.
3. Skinny is not the same as lean.
4. Minimize insulin surges by eating low GL foods (<150 g/day).
5. Think of milk as a source of sugar, not so much a source of protein.
6. Think of cheese as a condiment.
7. Protein satisfies hunger.
8. Eat healthy fat. Natural sources of Omega 3 are invaluable.
9. Eat considerably less beef, especially grain-fed beef.
10. Make better choices more often, not perfect choices all the time.

CHAPTER II

EXERCISE SCIENCE and SLEEP

"The secret to getting ahead is getting started."

Agatha Christie

Introduction to Exercise — Part I

"Every worthwhile accomplishment, big or little, has its stages of drudgery and triumph: a beginning, a struggle, and a victory."

Mahatma Gandhi

The Greatest Pill Ever

Exercise is perhaps the most effective and most thoroughly studied therapy we have found against chronic disease and ailments of age.

In women, for example, exercise during menopause reduces mortality, heart disease, osteoporosis, and protects cognition. Pelvic floor exercises specifically can improve satisfaction with sex and reduce urinary incontinence. As a point of perspective—exercise is known to reduce the risk of invasive breast cancer by 10% for each 4 hours of brisk walking per week. In men, exercise reduces mortality, heart disease, osteoporosis, and protects cognition as well. It is known to improve sexual activity, and is associated with a reduced incidence of prostate cancer.

Table 1.1

Three Major Domains Exercise Improves

Physical Domain
Muscle ▪ **Improved muscle strength, mass, power**
Bone ▪ Reduced osteoporosis ▪ Reduced fractures
Fat ▪ **Reduced body fat** ▪ Improved insulin sensitivity ▪ Improved fat use for fuel ▪ Reduced diabetes
Other ▪ Reduced vascular inflammation ▪ Improved wound healing and skin ▪ Reduced hypertension ▪ Improved integrity of ligaments, tendons, and joint function
Sexual Domain
▪ Reduced erectile dysfunction
Emotional Domain
▪ Improved energy and drive ▪ Reduced depressive mood ▪ Improved sense of well-being ▪ Improved concentration ▪ Improved sleep ▪ Reduced memory loss ▪ Reduced risk of dementia

The greatest pill, but the least used

Most of us know that diet and exercise are important to achieving and maintaining a healthy body. We are bombarded with media reports concerning health risks, exercise, foods, supplements, and the latest fads in fitness. Millions of dollars are spent yearly in the pursuit of fitness goals. Unfortunately, people tend to look for the quick fix or the shortcut that will magically transform their lifestyle into one that is healthier. As you probably already know, the results of these types of endeavors are usually less than advertised or are short-lived.

The quality of any exercise choice you make is highly dependent on what it is replacing.

We said something similar in the *Nutrition* chapter with respect to macronutrients. The same concept can be applied to exercise. At first, many are intimidated by the concept of daily intense exercise. That is to be expected. However, your body has an amazing capacity to adapt, especially when you start out slowly. We remind patients that any new exercise, however fit they may be, will be more taxing than they expect. The reason is essentially neurological. There are many factors that play into performance of exercise: cardiovascular fitness, strength, neuromuscular coordination specific to that sport, agility, flexibility, and balance (to name a few). Psychological components of exercise are very important as well, and often less accounted for when patients start new exercises or events. You may be fit and have an excellent VO_2 max that reflects a solid heart health, but if you are taking on a new athletic activity it might be harder than you expect. When you are familiar with the stresses associated with an exercise or event, you can concentrate on performance. You can anticipate when you need to push and when you can ease off the gas pedal. We call this the familiarity factor. When the familiarity is not present, you can expect at least a 20%–50% lower performance than you might predict for your fitness level. The point is to lower your expectations of your performance for the first few weeks or months of a new sport or exercise. The performance will come when you become more familiar with what to expect and when to expect it.

Like any journey, beginning an exercise routine is a stepwise process that, when made diligently and consistently, gets you to where you want to be.

Almost nobody starts out with daily intense exercise. The first step is to capitalize on what you do already. If you are not doing anything, getting off the couch into a weekly class that interests you can be a great start. If you are already into walking, Zumba, Tai Chi, or like to dance the Rumba, keep at it but progressively add resistance and aerobic training. Work with your care provider and a personal trainer to develop a program around your interests.

As we discuss later in the chapter, begin making changes by creating a pattern of **regular exercise**, whatever exercise you choose. Aim for 3–4 days a week, but make it regular. Find a time on certain days you like to work out and set that aside. One hour each session is ideal, but if you can only spare 30 minutes, it will be productive. Once you establish regularity each week, even if you start at once a week, steadily increase to daily workouts. They do not have to be intense, just daily. We believe it is a good idea to have one of your days a light/recovery day but that does not mean you should be inactive. That might be a good day to stretch, do balance exercises, or light walking/cycling. Once you establish **daily exercise**, you have made it through one of the biggest obstacles we see patients struggle with: scheduling. From a daily exercise pattern you will want to slowly increase your intensity. The bottom line is to slowly ramp up the frequency of **intense exercise**. You might start by choosing 1 day a week for an intense workout and adding another day in 2–4 weeks. The point is to continue to add regular intense workouts until you are able to do them daily. For some, this process may take as long as 1–2 years of committed progress to achieve **daily intense exercise.** That is ok. In fact, it is ok to take 3–4 years if you are really out of shape. Each week you make progress toward that goal, you are building your Banks. If you never reach daily intense exercise because it is not personally worth it to you, that is also ok. The "sweet spot" of how much work you do versus the returns is very personal. This chapter gives you all you need to know to go as far as you want with effective and beneficial exercise.

There is a lot of hard science that relates to fitness. There are specific ways to train for specific goals. Often times, people fail to maintain exercise programs because they simply don't see the type of results they were expecting. Sometimes this is due to what some might term as a lack of willpower or discipline. Many times, it is due to poor program design. That is, your exercise program simply cannot achieve the results you wish to see because it is designed to do something else. This is where the science comes in, and the science is something you can learn and understand. Once you do, you will be able to make intelligent decisions regarding your workouts. Whether you realize it or not, you have a lot of discipline. You exhibit it every day you go to work, take care of your kids, or tend to any of the hundreds of obligations you face as a part of your daily life. Applying this to a program of exercise and healthy eating is well within your capabilities. But we wouldn't expect you to put precious time and energy into something that doesn't work—we don't.

Focus on process goals, less on outcome goals

It is imperative that you know what your goals are in order to succeed in your fitness program. Only then can you proceed intelligently on your training program design. We strongly recommend investing in a personal trainer for the first 12 weeks. They will design a personalized program for you based on a sound *needs analysis*, including your interests and schedule. People who are new to the fitness lifestyle might not know much more than "I want to look better" or "I just want to get in shape." That's okay. Your trainer can guide you along at first, but picking the right trainer is important.

We explain to all of our patients the difference between outcome goals and process goals. For example, a worthwhile process goal is to train 5–6 days a week. An outcome goal is focused on specific, usually quantifiable, gains. For example, an outcome goal might be to gain 10 pounds of lean muscle tissue in 36 weeks. Placing value on process goals improves the probability that outcome goals are achieved; limits imposed by genetics or life events can interfere with outcome goals.

Process goals are within your scope of control. Outcome goals are not necessarily entirely within your scope of control.

As you improve your level of fitness, a whole new world of opportunities will be revealed to you. It is quite possible you will embark on activities you never thought you would be capable of doing. Your goals will change, and your program will change too. There are some important caveats to be aware of with respect to your goals. Often times, people have more than one goal in mind. In many instances, these goals might be incompatible with each other. That is, you can't train for both at the same time because they require different physiological adaptations and thus, different training programs. Often, people have preconceived notions of the type of exercise that they want to do. There may be nothing wrong with these approaches, but they might not be the ones that will help you achieve your goals. It is perhaps best to forget what you think you know, then learn the science of training, and then decide what you want to do. About 90% of all fitness programs are centered on a handful of basic principles. They simply must be adhered to at all times. You must learn and adhere to these principles if you want to be successful.

Exercise: Why one size doesn't fit all

As with nutrition, most people have a difficult time understanding exercise. This is not surprising, because most of the gurus talking about it don't seem to understand it either. That is not to say they don't know things about exercise, but rather, they don't understand exercise as a medical therapy.

Exercise is a prescription just like any other prescription. That means it is based upon one's individual needs. In exercise science, this is called a ***Needs Analysis***.

A *Needs Analysis* is much like the diagnostic tests a care provider performs when you go to hospital or clinic. Only after those tests are completed does the care provider recommend a treatment plan specific to your problem. You would think it totally absurd for your care provider to give you a treatment plan before he or she asked you what was wrong or examined you. Yet that is precisely what people do when it comes to exercise.

If we were writing an article for a men's magazine, our assumption would be that you are a 25-year-old urban male with no health problems or limitations. For a women's magazine, you would be a 30-year old suburban mom who wants to lose weight and "firm up". For an AARP blog, you would be a 55-year-old who is horribly unfit and incapable of mustering any real effort. So we tell the young man to do Crossfit, the women to do the Brazil Butt Lift and the 55-year old to walk briskly. What we recommend might be sound advice, but not necessarily appropriate for you, because the assumptions we made might be wrong.

That is why **your** exercise prescription must be based upon a *Needs Analysis* just like your nutrition prescription. The *Needs Analysis* considers your medical problems, exercise experience, time commitment, access to equipment, personal preferences, and specific goals. The prescription then must prioritize your goals and select the exercises best suited to achieving those goals.

As time passes, the program will vary if the objectives change. Even if the objectives don't change, the volume and intensity must vary to keep progressing.

This is a fundamental flaw people make when approaching exercise: a lack of a quality *Needs Analysis*. Following are four additional flaws in our perceptions about exercise.

The Four Biggest Misconceptions About Exercise

1. You get thin by exercising. *False*

Truth: Weight loss comes from intentionally reducing how much you eat. It takes conscious effort. Without the deliberate act of limiting how much we eat, we strongly tend to consume enough calories to stay the same weight. We learned this in the *Nutrition* chapter. Your mind has a way of controlling your appetite to maintain a set-point of weight. To reset the set-point, you have to be the boss of your brain. You have to say "No" until you retrain the brain to a new set-point. It takes effort.

Without the deliberate effort to eat less, you will eat enough food to compensate for the energy you use during exercise.

2. Exercise duration is more important than exercise intensity. *False*

Truth: If you are going to exercise to improve cardiovascular health, you will need to exercise at a relatively high level of intensity. As with resistance training, in which progressive overload leads to gains in strength, high heart rate, high-intensity interval training (HIIT) is a way of significantly improving cardiovascular health.

3. Weight lifting is only for body builders. *False*

Truth: Those who learn how to lift weights properly (resistance training) and train regularly will be most likely to be independent at 100 years of age. No guarantees are made about anything at that age, least of all the strength to get out of a chair or the ability to walk to the backyard. However we know that those skills are best developed in people who regularly exercise to increase quadriceps muscle strength, coordination, flexibility and balance.

> ***Quadriceps strength is the single greatest predictor of independence in the elderly.***

Other benefits of resistance training include slowing osteoporosis and keeping muscles toned. It's hard to do that without weights. The weights do not have to be the kind you see in in magazines, not at all. In fact, we would say that "glamorized" level of weight lifting probably is counterproductive as you age. If you are going to lift more than 1.5 times your weight, do it in your twenties. By the time we hit our forties, resistance training should be structured for being able to lift what you can lift 12–16 times, which is not a very heavy weight. Properly performed squats (with a bar and weights, with your butt going lower than your knees) will reduce the rate of muscle and bone loss (osteoporosis). Maintaining the musculoskeletal system will help significantly in maintaining your independence.

A well-rounded resistance-training program always includes squats. Men need to focus less on the chest, arms, and shoulders. At our age, it's time to get functional about our workouts. Big chests and arms don't help keep you independent and very well can land you in the surgeon's chair for an ineffective rotator cuff repair. Women should try to forget about who's watching whom at the gym and do what keeps you spritely and mobile. Weightlifting, especially squats, is irreplaceable.

4. Long, slow, distance (aerobic) training is the preferred method to train. *Not really true*

Training with HIIT training (anaerobic training) strengthens your heart. The first thing we tell relatively healthy patients is to get a baseline VO_2 max test done and start training with HIIT. With 12–20 minutes of hard workouts, 4 times a week, your heart will become healthier—faster than training with long distances at a slow pace.Low-intensity training does not help you much. It might burn a few more calories, but we already showed you why that won't affect how thin you are. The calories burned tend to be made up later by eating more. You have to stretch your limits to improve. The way the heart stretches is by getting close to your maximum heart rate. The bottom line is that running at a slow pace for long periods of time might be counterproductive.

Moderate periods of aerobic cardiovascular training can improve your heart health, but not nearly as efficiently as HIIT training.

Since your heart health is directly related to how long you live (we know this from hundreds of studies), you are better off training with low-volume HIIT.

Heart health can be measured with a test (usually on a bike) called VO_2 max. Those who have the highest (top 20th) percentile VO_2 max have about a 6% chance of dying in the next 10 years. Those in the lowest (bottom 20th) percentile have about a 25% of dying in the same 10-year period. You can change your VO_2 max with 80 minutes per week of HIIT training. Those who go from the bottom 20th to the next level reduce their chance of death by 50%.

Your body as a bank

Exercise contributes substantially to building your assets. It is especially helpful in reducing the debt of inflammation, which robs you of your efforts to build your assets. Exercise reduces inflammation by reducing body fat (assuming a sound nutritional program) and by producing anti-inflammatory agents that circulate throughout the body. Interleukin 6 (IL-6) is the most important of those agents. As we age, we become less effective in all systems, including our response to exercise. The earlier you start building your assets, the more you can work on maintaining them rather than trying to build them up.

The Banks

Building the Heart Bank

- VO_2 max naturally diminishes with age. Efforts to improve it go along way toward heart health

Building the Bone Bank

- Resistance exercise is very powerful in shoring up the Bone Bank
- Use weights, especially when you squat
- Running, as opposed to cycling, can also help improve your Bone Bank

Building the Muscle Bank

- Resistance exercises are essential to building your Muscle Bank
- Use weights, especially when you squat.
- As you get older, your quadriceps strength is directly related to your ability to stay out of a nursing home. Keep the quads strong.
- Focus on lower extremities and less on upper extremities

Build the Brain Bank

- Exercise's contribution to your Brain Bank is not proven. It certainly won't hurt it.

Types of Training and Tests — Part II

Introduction

B*efore we jump into the different types of exercises, it is important to review a few basic points of anatomy and physiology. We'll keep it brief.*

Basic Science Review

Muscle fiber types

Train your muscles for your sport or activity

There are two major types of muscle fibers, with an additional type that can serve as a transition muscle fiber.

Type I muscle fibers are often referred to as "slow twitch." They are the dominant fiber in long-distance runners. These fibers can use a lot of oxygen (aerobic respiration; Krebs cycle) to create energy, but doing this takes more time. They create less force than type II muscle fibers, but are efficient and can operate for a long time. They are easy to turn on and are hardy muscle fibers.

Type II muscle fibers are often referred to as "fast twitch." They are the dominant fiber in sprinters, and use less oxygen than type I fibers. Instead, they get most of their energy from faster-acting sources, running out of fuel much more quickly than type 1 fibers. They generate a lot of force, but are prone to fatigue and injury. Type II fibers take more electrical impulses from the nervous system to turn on than type I muscle fibers.

The third type of muscle fiber we will share with you is the type IIx fiber. Technically, it is one of the fastest we have. It can be used as a type II fiber, for quick action activities, but it also serves as a fiber that can be transformed into type I. When a cell can become one type of cell or another, we say it has the potential for many cell types (pluripotent). Type IIx fibers are considered pluripotent. With training, a small percentage of muscle fibers that are type IIx can become type I.

Energy systems

Which one does your sport or activity use the most?

There are three major types of energy systems muscle fibers use. They range from super-fast to slow. All of the systems produce energy by releasing the energy that is held in the bond between phosphate and other molecules. All cells have the capacity to use any of the systems, but one system is usually preferred, based on the other cell components. Specific molecules are needed to break the phosphate bonds to release energy. We call molecules that make reactions like that *enzymes.*

The super-fast energy system is called the phosphocreatine system, but it only provides a few seconds' worth of energy. The next level of quick access energy is through a process that does not need oxygen (anaerobic glycolysis). It can produce energy for about two minutes before it runs out. The slowest, but most efficient, energy system is called respiration (using aerobic glycolysis and the Krebs cycle). As you already know, respiration requires oxygen.

Type I muscle fibers use oxygen. Type II muscle fibers tend to use the faster but less efficient systems, but some slower fibers (of the type II muscle fibers) still use respiration to a lesser degree than type I muscle fibers.

Figure 2.1

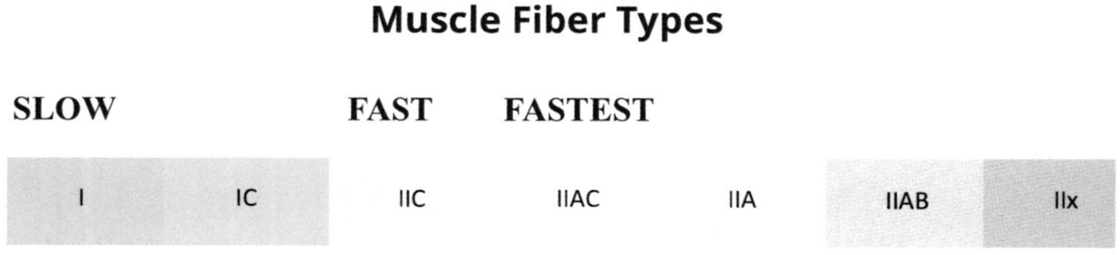

Muscle Fiber Types

SLOW FAST FASTEST

I IC IIC IIAC IIA IIAB IIx

Power, Strength, Hypertrophy & Muscular Endurance

Which one does your sport or activity use the most?

Resistance training generally involves 3–4 classifications of training: muscular endurance, hypertrophy (growth), strength, and power. Conceptually, these classifications can be thought of as a spectrum, similar to the idea that metabolic systems are found in a spectrum. The two major variations are how fast the movement is and how long the movements can be sustained. In a way, these variables reflect the kind of muscle fibers being used.

In all resistance exercises, elements of muscular endurance, hypertrophy, strength, and power contribute to executing the exercise, but one dominates depending on the action.

Power exercises are performed over a short interval (≤2 seconds) and are often considered high-velocity forms of strength. Sometimes power is referred to as "fast strength." Only a couple of repetitions can be performed before exhaustion. A longer recovery is also needed compared with exercises that involve endurance.

Strength exercises are performed over slightly longer intervals compared with power exercises, generally 3–5 seconds. Only a few repetitions can be performed at near maximum strength.

Hypertrophy is performed at much higher repetitions than either power or strength. Only around 60% of maximum strength (sometimes less) is used for hypertrophy exercises.

Local muscular endurance (LME) endurance is associated with even higher repetitions than hypertrophy. LME is typically used for training athletes whose sport requires multiple repetitive actions under fatigue (cyclists).

All repetitions of the above resistance exercises are derived from the maximum you can lift, one time (1RM). Typically a maximum squat and bench press are used to create the amount of weight (load) you will lift and how many times you will lift it (repetitions). The load and repetition will vary according to whether you are aiming for power, strength, hypertrophy, or LME gains. If you are relatively new to lifting weights, your trainer might establish a 3-repetition maximum (3RM) instead of a 1RM, because it will be a more reliable number. The formulas used to derive the loads from a 3RM are adequate for a novice weight lifter.

Table 2.1

Load/Intensity vs. Adaptation with Resistance Training

Goal	Load (% 1RM)	Goal Repetitions
Power	80–90	1–5
Strength	>85	<6
Hypertrophy	67–85	6–10
Muscular endurance	<67	>12

Adapted from Baechle et al.

Flexibility

Focus on days off and after workouts

Flexibility is perhaps the most commonly neglected element of exercise we need to develop and maintain as we get older. Flexibility is very important in staying independent and staying out of a nursing home. Furthermore, imbalances in flexibility can contribute to chronic pain conditions well before nursing home status.

Flexibility can be performed on days off during your weekly exercise schedule. The most important thing to remember is that your body should be awake and warm when you work on flexibility. Slow progression with limited discomfort is a much smarter approach than trying to make too much progress too fast. Starting on flexibility training during middle age (if not sooner) is a smarter approach than waiting until you are elderly.

Balance

Takes seconds to train, and can save you from a fall later in life

Balance skills can be developed later in life, but are most influenced by activities before 10 years of age. Like flexibility, balance becomes increasingly important in staying independent as you age.

There are two types of balance. Balance when moving (like on a bike) is called dynamic balance. Static balance dictates the patient's ability to control their center of gravity over their base of support. Good balance of both types is central to preventing falls and fractures.

It takes very little time to work on balance. Try closing your eyes and lifting one foot a few inches off the ground. Do both sides. You'll usually find one side is much better than the other. Even 15 seconds can be challenging. Work on this daily until you can balance for 30 seconds or more on each leg. It takes less than 5 minutes a day, and might ultimately save you from a fall. In addition, squats and other compound lower extremity exercises will sharpen the nervous system and the small muscles in the feet, which can contribute significantly to improved balance.

Endurance

Endurance is a general word that is used to describe any force, speed, or metabolic action over an extended period of time. Time is the key element that distinguishes endurance.

- Strength endurance is the limit of strength that can be generated over time.
- Speed endurance is the maximum speed that can be generated over time.
- Local muscular endurance is the submaximal force that can be generated over time.
- Cardiopulmonary endurance is the maximum capacity to provide oxygen and remove waste products over time.

For aging patients, local muscular endurance can be important because it tests your muscles' capacity to perform repeated tasks, like walking or picking up objects. Successful performance of such tasks can make the difference between independent living and disability. Local muscular endurance primarily affects the type I muscle fibers, or slow twitch fibers. Local muscular endurance techniques are often the cornerstone of functional strength-building programs.

Principles of Exercise and Training

Part III

*I*n this section we share common and useful training principles that you and your trainer will want to use to create an individualized exercise program. Perhaps the most important applied principles to understand are the Progressive and the Overload principles (often cited together). We cover those and others below.

Stress - GAS (General Adaptation Syndrome)

Hans Selye coined the phrase "only the dead have no stress."

> ***Stress is required to grow, but not all stress promotes growth. Good stress promotes growth, and bad stress is destructive.***

The GAS principle describes the stages of adapting to stress. First, your body signals an alarm (overload). Second, your body adapts by responding with resistance (overcompensation). Finally, if the stress is too much, the body exhausts its reserves and begins to enter an overtraining state. Overtraining can lead to losses in strength or speed and can reduce your motivation to train. Avoid overtraining, but don't mistake a lactate burn in the legs or gasping for air for overtraining. Those experiences are typical for any training program.

With rest, after resistance, you rebuild. *Rest is essential.*

A - Adaptation
R - Resistance
E - Exhaustion

Overload Principle

Each workout session and training cycle needs to create mild overload. The overload principle states that training must include higher levels of stress than the body is accustomed to. Ideally, overload involves eustress (good stress), rather than distress (bad stress). Careful awareness of overtraining helps to keep overload a positive stressor.

Overload can come in the form of increasing the weight (load), the number of times you lift the weight (repetitions), the number of sets (groups of repetitions) or reducing the amount of rest between sets. Also, varying the exercises slightly can create a type of overload by reducing the adaptation (we discussed above). The mind and body are amazingly efficient and able to adapt, but for growth purposes we want limited adaptation. Some people have referred to these variations in exercises as "muscle confusion," which is a handy way to describe it.

Progressive Principle

The intensity of workouts should increase as you train. The progressive principle is very closely related to the overload principle. It states that the load or stress must continue to increase to promote adaptive increases in strength, speed, or another variable being trained. Very often, progressive overload is described as a single principle.

Progressive overload leads to overreaching. Overreaching is what you need to do to create gain—go briefly beyond your expected limit. However overreaching, if done too often, will lead to overtraining.

Specific Adaptations to Imposed Demands (SAID)

The body is adept at becoming efficient

The SAID principle states that the body adapts in a very specific way based on the specific stress. You become efficient with that specific exercise.

This principle is central to athletes improving their strength or speed. A training program will often include specific resistance exercises that mimic the specific skills you execute in your sport. These types of exercises are referred to as sport-specific training.

Overtraining

Rest is critical to making progress

Overtraining is an athlete's physical and emotional response to training that is too intense. Overtraining comes after overreaching too often or too long. As we said, you want to overreach—bite off more than you can sometimes.

> ***You don't want to overreach all the time or you will collapse. But make no mistake, without overreaching, you will not improve your cardiovascular fitness or strength.***

Initially, hard training causes underperformance. As you resist the stress, you overcompensate. Overcompensation that is followed by brief rest leads to rebuilding. It can be thought of as improving the castle walls under siege, before the walls collapse. The alarm is the attack on the castle, the resistance is not allowing the walls to fall. With a respite in the attack, the team in the castle can regroup and strengthen that wall, sometimes pulling resources from other places in the castle. Your body is the castle. Overcompensation followed by rest lets you keep the castle going.

If you don't allow yourself to rest, which may vary in length of time according to the initial force, you will not be able to rebuild. Instead, you enter into overtraining, finding yourself becoming weaker and less fit.

Therefore, your training program will be designed to avoid overtraining. You will want to maximize overreaching because that leads to building through overcompensation. We call this program design, when scheduled over a year or more, a *Periodized Program*. We will discuss this shortly.

> ***Aging patients are especially prone to overtraining because they require more time for recovery.***

It is just the way it is. As a general rule, 50% more time for recovery is commonly required for a middle-aged athlete compared with an athlete in their 20s.

Being aware of the common signals your body sends during overtraining is valuable.

You can check for lymphadenopathy by placing your fingers where we find lymph nodes: the neck, groin, and armpits.

Your performance during HIIT training will tell you if you are entering overtraining because you will not be able to perform as many intervals for as long as you have been able to in the past.

You should always check your heart rate recovery after working out. Your heart rate should recover at least 12 beats per minute within the first minute of ending your last interval. You can still move during that minute, but not forcefully. Once you get into the routine of checking your heart rate after intense exercise, you will automatically notice when it is not recovering as quickly, because your post-interval routine is similar each time.

Your resting pulse rate will commonly drop once you start training, particularly if training is new to you. It might only drop a few beats per minute. Once you have a consistent resting heart rate, you can monitor it for an uptick if you suspect overtraining. This has become more convenient because wearable devices can now give you personal data on a daily, if not minute-to-minute basis.

You might also notice other signs of stress, like more sweating for no apparent reason.

Symptoms of overtraining overlap with other stress-induced conditions. Early symptoms include reduced sleep quality and/or length of time. Depression and a sense of fatigue are also relatively common. Later, weight loss and emotional volatility might be evident.

If you suspect overtraining, it is best to rest. There is no rush. The benefits of exercise are lifetime, but you have to stay in the game to reap those rewards. Overtraining risks not only losing hard-won gains, but might demotivate you from training altogether. As you become more experienced (and in touch with your body) you will begin to know the fine line between overreaching and overtraining. Until then, it is much better to err on the side of resting and recovering, than risk overtraining.

A note on personal trainers

Get one—a good one

We believe strongly that everyone needs a coach, or a team of coaches, to navigate all components of health, including nutrition and exercise. This need is especially true for beginning- and intermediate-level athletes. Even elite athletes need coaches.

As with any coach you choose, picking the right one may be critical to the success or failure of your efforts. There is no recipe for a great coach, but we can share with you the qualities we often see. We encourage you to diligently screen before you commit time, money and effort into your program. A great coach will be an invaluable asset, but few are great.

At the very least, all coaches or personal trainers should start with a Needs Analysis. The Needs Analysis is an information gathering process (before you start working out) whereby your potential coach establishes your goals, your training level and will start to formulate a plan—a plan for you.

Basic nutritional tenets should be part of their discussion with you, and those tenets should sound familiar after reading the *Nutrition* chapter.

The plan they create for you should include a periodized program, which lays out the months ahead and what specific exercises you will be doing. The periodized program should include progressive overload principles and specific rest days. The program will likely be adjusted as your coach gets to know you better in the weeks ahead.

Good coaches walk the walk. They are fit and healthy. They are rarely late. They often do not tolerate clients who are late. Good coaches will be positive and will respect your limits.

The best coaches look for clients who come to sessions on time, come well rested, and do their best to stick to a good nutritional plan during training.

Adaptations to Training — Part IV

Introduction

*A*daptations to training are the keystone to gains or growth. In order to promote adaptations, **stress must be followed by rest.** We know you have read this already, but it is worth repeating. Additionally, the stresses must vary. The body is amazing at its capacity to adapt. It also has an amazing ability to conserve energy (store fat). We are constantly benefited by the former and thwarted by the latter.

Adaptation occurs by applying a stress or training stimulus. Five general areas of adaptation include the musculoskeletal, bioenergetics/metabolism, neurological, endocrine, and cardiorespiratory systems. With adaptation comes a leveling of performance (plateau) that must be challenged to allow continued gains. In the aging patient, effort is required to maintain those plateaus or prevent decline.

Musculoskeletal Fibers

Do you use slow- or fast-twitch muscle fibers in your activity?

Training induces structural and bioenergetic/metabolic changes in your muscle fibers. The individual muscle fibers get bigger (hypertrophy) with training. In addition, there can be more connections between the muscle fibers (crosslinking). Both of these adaptations make you faster and stronger.

Muscle fibers differ according to their force generation capacity, primary metabolic cellular systems used, fatigue potential, injury potential, and neural input required to activate (recruitment potential).

The kind of training you do dictates what muscle fibers (and systems) are activated. This is why if you want to train for a long-distance run, but have been sprinting all year, you will need to give your body time to adjust the energy systems, muscle fiber types (to a limited degree), and other cellular processes, to maximize their efficiency during a long-distance run. The transition that an athlete undertakes when they change the type of sport or event they are training for can be substantial. Patience is required to allow your body to make those changes so you can be efficient.

Table 4.1

Training Program Type According to Muscle Fiber Type

Athlete	Fiber Type Desired	Training Program Type with Mix of Volume/Intensity
Aerobic-Endurance	Type I	Resistance and endurance using high-volume, low-intensity plus HIIT
Anaerobic-Power	Type II	Resistance using high-intensity, low-volume, high-velocity

Adapted from Wilson et al.

Metabolic Adaptations (Energy Systems in the Cell)

Which energy system does your activity use the most?

Your muscle cells have enough stored adenosine triphosphate (ATP) to contract for just 1.26 seconds.. To replace the used ATP, your muscle cell must have glucose and be able to break it down rapidly. Muscles store glucose in stacks called glycogen. We have already discussed the three major energy systems used to turn sugar into energy: phosphocreatine, glycolysis (which can be done with and without oxygen), and respiration (which requires oxygen).

Depending on the muscle cell type (I or II), one of the three systems is used more in the cell, but all three are accessible. You can train your muscle cell to use more of one type of energy system or another by doing exercises that demand that system (based on speed of access and regeneration of the energy). If you sprint, your muscle cells will adapt to have the cellular machinery in place to accommodate the sprinting effort. If you run long distances, your cellular machinery will switch to adapt to that, though it might take several weeks to notice the increased efficiency. The adaptability of your metabolic systems is one of many examples that highlight the need to know how to train to your specific goals.

Lactate

Onset of blood lactate accumulation (OBLA): When lactate starts to move out of your muscles into your bloodstream

Lactate is the by-product of anaerobic energy production. Typically, you will create energy by cellular respiration (with oxygen). Using oxygen allows you make a lot more energy in the cell than without it. There are other ways to generate energy in a cell when you cannot deliver enough oxygen fast enough. One way is by breaking the creatine-phosphate bond, releasing energy. The creatine phosphate is sitting in your muscle cells ready to be used, but only a limited amount is present. The other way is through glycolysis. Glycolysis can occur with or without oxygen. When oxygen is not available, only a limited amount of energy is made. Lactate builds up in the muscle cell because it is a by-product of energy production when no oxygen is present (anaerobic). Lactate will stop further energy production, so it needs to be removed from the muscle cell. It usually gets transported out of the muscle, into the blood, and to the liver where it is recycled, so to speak. We can measure the blood levels of lactate pretty easily using a small finger prick. We know that when someone starts building up lactate in their blood, they are reaching their limit of work ability. The onset of blood lactate accumulation (OBLA) is an important marker in training. You can train so that you delay when this occurs, improving your body's ability to use oxygen. This is important in any athletic activity.

Lactate concentration, threshold, and VO_2 max

The typical concentration of lactate in the blood at rest is 0.5–2.2 mmol/L.The typical concentration of lactate after working hard (to fatigue) is >20 mmol/L.

As you now know, OBLA is a term used to describe a point during exercise when the blood lactate levels begin to rise significantly, either from increased production or reduced clearance. A commonly used number for OBLA is approximately 4 mmol/L. However, each individual is different. OBLA testing is often used in training to determine progressive workout programs to increase efficient processing of lactate, which results in increased power.

Your lactate threshold is reflected to a strong degree in the VO_2 max test you might take at the beginning of a program. Where VO_2 max uses heart rate as the marker for cardiovascular stress, lactate threshold testing uses the build up of lactate in the blood as a measure of cardiovascular stress. They are related, but not the same. Lactate threshold testing is more precise for competitive athletes who need to maximize their gains during their limited training periods.

In the trained athlete, the lactate threshold often falls between 70%–80% of their VO2 max. In the untrained athlete the lactate threshold often falls between 50%–60% of VO2 max.

This is why when you start to workout from an unconditioned state, it hurts so much so early. Don't let that dissuade you from showing up again and again. Your physiology will change. Give it time. The maximum lactate steady state (MLSS) is considered by some experts to be an even better indicator of aerobic capacity than VO_2 max. The MLSS might be a better marker for cardiovascular health. However, it requires a 40-minute testing period and multiple lactate samples (pin prick of the finger) during the exam.

Factors that influence lactate levels include intensity of exercise, the training status of the athlete, muscle fiber type, and initial muscle cell stored sugar (glycogen) levels. More intense exercises lead to higher levels of lactate. A well-trained athlete will have lower levels of lactate for similar workloads than less-trained athletes, but will be able to achieve higher levels of lactate because they are well trained and are able to work at higher levels of intensity. Type II muscle fibers generate more lactate for a given workload compared with type I muscle fibers. The more glycogen the muscle cell has to begin with, the higher the potential intensity, and also the higher the lactate levels that will be achieved.

> ***If you start a workout session depleted of glycogen (not fully recovered or not eating properly), you will have a less effective workout because the muscle cells will not have enough energy to perform.***

Aerobic training promotes hypertrophy of type I fibers and stimulates conversion from type II to type IIx to promote efficient aerobic metabolism. Type IIx fibers are more flexible and can ultimately be converted into type I fibers. Type I fibers tend to use less glycogen and more fat for metabolism, resulting in less lactic acid and lactate formation. Thus, the lactate threshold or OBLA is delayed. This adaptation allows the athlete to perform at higher percentage of their VO_2 max for longer. Once lactate starts to form, the exercise (or competition) has limited time remaining.

Low-volume, high-intensity interval training (HIIT) benefits include increased VO_2 max, increased muscle oxidative potential, buffering capacity (to neutralize lactate), and glycogen content. Hormonal changes that you will see with HIIT include a transient increase in cortisol, growth hormone, and testosterone. Body fat reduction with HIIT training is potentially high due to excess post-exercise oxygen consumption (EPOC).

Excess post exercise oxygen consumption

Continue burning energy into tomorrow to rebuild from a workout

EPOC refers to the observed continued increased calorie burning associated with anaerobic HIIT training, far more so than continuous aerobic training. Calories continue to burn well after the HIIT training, sometimes as long as 38 hours after the training session. This is why you might be starving the day after a workout, even if you aren't training that day. The body continues to work to return to a homeostatic resting state. Oxygen is the preferred fuel to get that work done. So, your cellular oxygen consumption continues until each cell is restored to full glycogen storage and has refitted the mitochondria for your next bout of work. As we age, this repair process takes more time. Testosterone helps your body in the repair process as well. Among many other deteriorating systems as we age, low testosterone is one of the reasons we need more time to recover.

Neurologic Adaptations

Often the first system to adapt to new training

Muscle contraction begins with an electrical signal from a motor nerve. Each motor nerve innervates a number of motor units ranging from a few (ocular) to many (quadriceps). When a motor nerve successfully signals a motor unit, the entire unit contracts.

Successful signaling a motor unit is called recruitment. When recruitment occurs, all fibers contract fully. Power is a reflection of the number of recruited motor units. Different motor units comprised of different muscle fiber types have different recruitment potential.

Generally, but not always, lower threshold units are recruited first.. Type I are considered lower threshold compared to type II muscle fibers. With higher motor neuron stimulus, more type II fibers are recruited. Low resistance exercises will use more type I muscle fibers, whereas heavier resistance exercises will demand more type II muscle fibers.

By exercising a muscle through a variety of angles and actions, a maximum number of motor units might be recruited, which is known as the "muscle confusion principle."

Endocrine Adaptations: Testosterone, Cortisol, IGF

Your hormones love when you exercise

Exercise (and other stress) creates complex hormonal responses. Changes include increases in the absolute amount of the hormone, receptors that become more sensitive, or slower removal of the hormones (clearance). The above changes will increase the effect of the hormone. Anaerobic training programs are known to increase testosterone, growth hormone, and cortisol. The cortisol increase is usually transient.

Sustained aerobic exercise (for example, a 10k run) will show elevated cortisol and lower total testosterone, but a higher amount of free testosterone. The net effect is hard to measure, but sexual dysfunction in elite aerobic athletes is commonly reported.

Some of the hormone changes we can measure because they show up in the blood. Other effects we know happen because of lab studies, but we cannot measure them in a live person. One interesting and very powerful way that hormones affect your body is when they are made in the same cell they then act upon. This process of making a hormone that acts on the cell that made it is called an autocrine effect (instead of endocrine). It is not measurable and usually occurs at very local tissue level.

We discuss hormone changes you might experience with training in more detail below.

Testosterone

Testosterone is a hormone that we call anabolic—which means it builds tissue. Growth hormone and insulin are also anabolic.

Testosterone increases with anaerobic (resistance and HIIT) training. Specific resistance training exercises include those with compound movements (deadlifts, power clean, and squats). Heavier weights promote more testosterone secretion. Higher intensity exercises promote testosterone secretion, including those with short rest periods (<60 seconds), high volume, and multiple sets. The more experienced the athlete is at lifting, the more testosterone will be produced. We usually see this effect in athletes who have been training for more than 2 years. Increases in women are not reliably detected, but might be due to the low baseline level, serum assay detection limits, and hemoconcentration effects.

Testosterone further promotes growth hormone (GH) secretion. It promotes protein building and can act on neurons to promote neurotransmitter release. The organ with the most testosterone receptors is the brain.

Testosterone decreases with endurance training (aerobic). The mechanism is not clear, but endurance athletes often have low testosterone. It typically takes years to develop, but might dramatically impact sex drive.

Growth hormone

Growth hormone is another anabolic hormone. GH enhances amino acid uptake and protein synthesis in type I and II muscle fibers. Exercise and good sleep increase GH secretion.

GH injections do not result in measurable strength gains, though people often get "bigger" because of fluid retention.

Insulin like growth factor (IGF-1) is an indirect way of measuring GH. It is useful because measuring GH is not practical, but measuring IGF-1 is, because it has a very long half-life.

Insulin like growth factor

IGF-1 is a molecule that often works locally, similar to the autocrine effects we described above. It can act on the same cell that makes it (autocrine) or on local cells (paracrine). IGF-1 levels are known to be more sensitive to food intake before and after exercise, which explains why certain pre- and post-workout supplements that contain high quality protein and carbohydrates are recommended.

Cortisol

Cortisol is a catabolic hormone, which means it breaks tissue down. Resistance exercises of high intensity (high-volume, with short rest periods, or low-volume with heavy weights) result in cortisol elevation. Cortisol levels are directly correlated with anaerobic stimuli.

Heart Adaptations

Build your Heart Bank

Short duration HIIT training improves VO_2 max primarily through improved perfusion and removal of the byproducts of metabolism (CO_2 and lactate). Recall, HIIT training improves your cardiovascular function through anaerobic workouts.

Resistance training does not change VO_2 max, but it does add other benefits, like core and leg strength and balance. Such benefits reduce the chance of falls and fractures.

Aerobic training (long slow distances) results in increased VO_2 max, primarily through improving the heart's performance. The heart becomes better at pumping more blood on each stroke (increased stroke volume). With improved pumping, your heart rate then can decrease because enough blood is being delivered to the tissues. At the level of the muscle cell, adaptations make them more efficient at using oxygen (respiration). Over 6–12 months, improvements in these cellular functions will delay the time that lactate shows up in the blood (OBLA). Improvements may occur for years with consistent training.

Exercise effects on heart disease risk

Heart disease risk is reduced considerably with exercise

One way we measure your cardiovascular health is to see how well your blood vessels dilate. Flexible blood vessels are healthy blood vessels. They dilate with increased work or exercise. As flow through them increases, they dilate (flow mediated dilation, or FMD). With age, the natural course is for those blood vessels to become less flexible (and they often develop atherosclerotic plaques). So, with age, FMD will decrease. People who regularly exercise retain the flexibility of their blood vessels.

Along the same lines, we can measure the carotid artery to see how well it responds to increased flow with exercise. We use ultrasound to determine the compliance of the carotid artery. The better the compliance, the healthier the blood vessel. We know that with as little as three months of exercise, carotid artery compliance improves significantly.

The overweight and obese typically have higher lipoprotein levels (LDL and VLDL) than normal weight individuals. They also have more oxidized lipoproteins. Oxidized LDL and VLDL are more likely to cause damage to blood vessels. Thus, the overweight and obese have more damaging LDL and VLDL than those of normal weight. With exercise, however, the overweight can reduce their levels of the oxidized lipoproteins to a similar ratio that we see in normal weight individuals. So even if they don't lose weight, the exercise reduces lab markers of cardiovascular risk (oxidized lipoproteins are worse than regular lipoproteins).

We know that those who exercise show around a 40% improvement in all lab markers related to cardiovascular disease. More importantly, we also know that those who exercise more than 1500 kcal per week have a 60% reduction in cardiovascular disease-related clinical events, such as heart attacks. So the lab marker improvements actually underestimate how much improvement you make to your health with 1500 kcal of training each week.

To put that amount of calories into perspective, a solid HIIT session of 4–6 intervals over a 20-minute period will burn about 400 kcal, depending on the specific effort. Therefore, around 4 training sessions per week substantially improves your cardiovascular health. This outcome is consistent with other studies that show 3–4 HIIT trainings per week improve cardiovascular health, though those studies did not measure calories burned.

Anti-Inflammatory Effects of Exercise

Part V

Introduction

*I*n the past, humans used to move a lot more. Daily walking and energy expenditure during work was the norm for most people. Today, the need to move has been replaced, by some, with regular structured exercise sessions. We hope everyone recognizes the need to move daily. Not every day needs to be an intense workout session. It cannot be.

> ***Recognizing the body's (and mind's) need to be fully engaged in the world around it is critical in an increasingly virtual world, where movement is not required.***

As with weight loss, a deliberate effort needs to be made to accommodate the lack of physical activity required of us today. That is not to say exercise leads to weight loss. We know in the end, exercise does not lead to significant weight loss without deliberately eating less. We are simply saying that intentional effort is required to counter an environment that promotes a sedentary lifestyle. Our genes have a long way to go before they adapt to the much faster changes in lifestyle. Recognizing we still need to be active is important to our long-term health. One area of great interest is how integral inflammation is to our modern lives and how well exercise combats inflammation.

Inflammation is an underlying cause of many chronic diseases, including heart disease. Specifically to aging, inflammation causes cardiovascular disease, the #1 cause of death worldwide. We discuss how this happens in the *Nutrition* and the *Hormone Replacement* chapters. But we want to remind you that cardiovascular disease is neither caused by eating too much fat nor by clogged arteries. Increased inflammation has also been correlated with cancer (breast and colon), type II diabetes mellitus (DMII), Alzheimer's dementia, depression, hypertension, obsessive compulsive disorder, rheumatologic disease, inflammatory bowel disease, and others. Such diseases can be characterized as the cluster of diseases related to physical inactivity.

Figure 5.1

Diseases Associated with Increased Inflammation

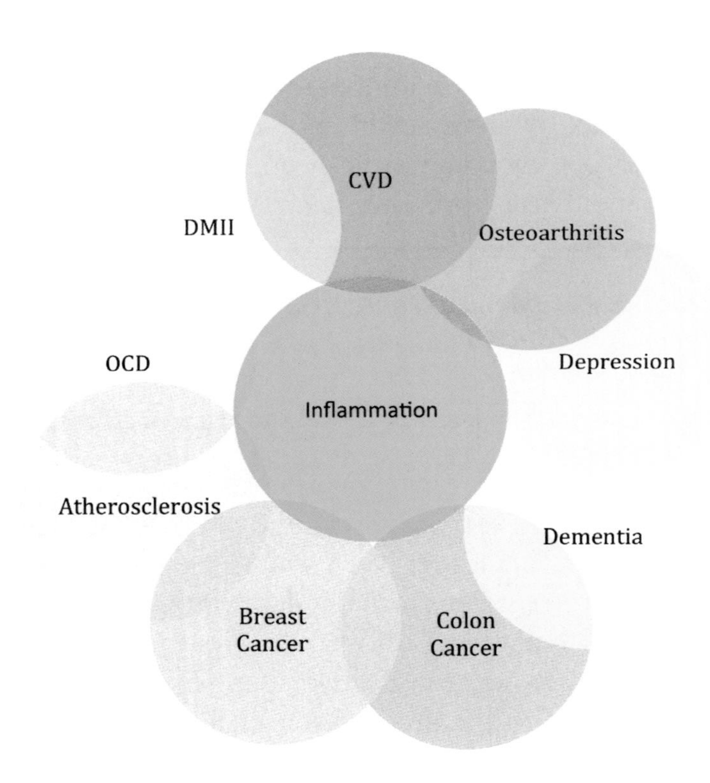

Adapted from Pedersen

The benefits of exercise in reducing inflammation are impressive. If you want to reduce the untoward effects of inflammation, which we are all overexposed to in the contemporary world, exercise is the simplest and most effective way to do it. You can't beat the benefits of exercise, but the benefits are particularly powerful when it comes to reducing inflammation.

Muscle Is An Anti-Inflammatory Organ

As discussed in the *Nutrition* chapter, there are 3 main phases of inflammation: the vascular, cellular, and resolution phases.

Long-term, consistent exercise reduces inflammation. In large part, muscle acts as an endocrine organ. Muscle tissue contains specific anti-inflammatory molecules, called myokines, that reduce overall inflammation and work to resolve chronic unresolved inflammation. IL-6 is probably the most important inflammatory marker to know about when it comes to exercise.

In general, the higher the **intensity** of the exercise, the more you will create an anti-inflammatory environment. We stress intensity not because we want everyone to be stressed about exercise. On the contrary, we want everyone to embrace a little stress. Few trainers are willing to risk their client relationship by creating intense programs. In the end, many clients do not get the results they are looking for when they do not have the right path and the right intensity to create the changes they want. Your body will tell you when you are overtraining.

The duration of exercise is much less important than the intensity. Intense exercise results in a strong anti-inflammatory response by your muscles.

IL-6 has the potential as an anti-inflammatory or pro-inflammatory molecule, depending on the conditions that result in its formation. IL-6 increases caused by exercise are anti-inflammatory. In other conditions, like infection, IL-6 might promote inflammation because of other molecules like tumor necrosis factor alpha (TNFα). Thus, IL-6 can promote inflammation (sepsis) or suppress inflammation (exercise). It is currently thought the ratio of IL-6/TNFα is the determining factor of whether IL-6 is pro- or anti-inflammatory. When IL-6 is present without elevated TNFα, it is not only an anti-inflammatory agent but it promotes healthier metabolism (using fat instead of carbs). Exercise results in more fat burning and less fat storage. It reduces insulin resistance and improves appetite regulation.

Inflammatory adaptations with exercise

Exercise tends to reduce inflammation

Moderate exercise in young healthy adults has been shown to increase IL-6 by nearly 20 times. It works in the elderly as well. When you exercise substantially, you reduce the sugar stored in your muscle cells (glycogen). Low sugar stored in cells increases IL-6 production. In this way, IL-6 is thought to be a type of energy sensor.

> ***Carbohydrates blunt the production of IL-6 (an exercise-induced anti-inflammatory agent).***

Glycogen levels tend to be higher in trained athletes for two reasons: the trained athlete's metabolism has adapted to store more glycogen; and trained athletes have adapted to burn fat as a fuel, more so than the untrained athlete who tends to use up the stored glycogen quickly during exercise. Thus, glycogen levels tend to stay high in the trained athlete, compared with the untrained, for any given level of exercise. Because IL-6 production is highly dependent on glycogen stores in the muscle cell, the trained athlete requires more substantial exercise to reach the same levels of IL-6 compared with untrained athletes.

A concentric exercise is one in which the muscle shortens (such as triceps in the bench press). An eccentric exercise is one in which the muscle lengthens (hamstrings in certain phases of running). Eccentric exercises are thought to cause more stress and micro-damage to muscles. With appropriate protein intake, the repairs are easily made. We also know that eccentric exercises such as running or sprinting might have greater positive impact on inflammation. In part, this might contribute to the profoundly positive impact that we see with HIIT, especially if you choose sprinting as your mode of exercise.

VO_2 max and Evidence for Longevity

Part VI

Introduction

*T*raditionally, there are four vital signs: temperature, blood pressure, heart rate, and respiratory rate. VO_2 max, for all practical purposes, could be considered your fifth vital sign.

Studies in the past two decades have solidified the value of cardiovascular testing and how the performance on those tests impacts mortality. The better a person's cardiovascular capacity, the longer their lifespan. Following governmental or other agency recommendations on physical activity might not lead to improved cardiovascular capacity. Unfortunately, as we saw in the *Nutrition* chapter, government-recommended guidelines (of cardiovascular fitness levels) do not correlate with recommended physical activity levels that improve health. Those recommendations don't improve people's cardiovascular capacity. Don't buy the pie-in-the-sky dream that walking 3 times a week is going to create big changes for you. If you want to do something a few times a week, and have it not take up a lot of time, it is going to have to be an intense workout during those short periods. We'll talk about how you can invest as little as 80 minutes a week and see improvement in your projected lifespan. But we want to emphasize that you can do much more once you realize how much your body can adapt. You just have to show up, try hard, and give it time. The changes will come and the benefits are real.

How your cardiovascular fitness is attained, maintained, improved, and tested are important choices to make. When you go through your exercise testing (VO_2 max or MLSS), you might find out you are in the top quintile (top fifth of people your age and weight) or you might find out you have exercise intolerance. Invest the best effort you can to be sure that lack of effort is not the cause of poor test results. There is no failing or passing of the test, it is just a baseline from which to improve. Show up well rested and not hungry, but do not eat a full meal within 3 hours before the test. An apple or something easy to digest around an hour before the test is reasonable. Most of the time, you will be offered a bike VO_2 max test. But there are many ways to establish a baseline cardiovascular fitness, including a 12-minute run, treadmill, or even a stair climbing test. Whichever test you choose, be sure to use that in follow-up visits.

Exercise testing variables to know

Exercise heart rate

Provides data on cardiac output (CO=HR*SV), where HR is heart rate and SV is stroke volume. At submaximal workloads, the HR should remain relatively low because the SV usually picks up the bulk of the performance at low workloads in fit individuals. Aerobic training tends to improve cardiovascular health by first increasing the stroke volume; anaerobic HIIT training tends to work at the tissue level by improving O_2 delivery and waste removal efficiency.

HRR

Heart rate reserve (HRR) is the difference between your maximum heart rate and your recovery heart rate at 1 minute. An HRR <12 bpm is considered abnormal. However, it is important to consider context when measuring recovery. If you are deconditioned, the HRR will be slower. If you are working out for a long period of time, the HRR might also be slower.

Exercise BP

Diastolic blood pressure should remain stable during exercise. For men, the systolic blood pressure might increase up to 210 mmHg and for women up to 190 mmHg and be considered normal responses.

EKG

Exercise does not change your normal sinus rhythm.

Pulse Oximetry

Pulse oximetry should not change with exercise. If it is $\leq$95%, it might reflect interstitial lung disease.

VO_2 max (absolute)

The absolute volume of oxygen consumed during your workout. The units are in liters per minute.

VO_2 max (relative)

VO_2 max provides data on aerobic fitness, as we have discussed. It measures the cardiac output and volume of oxygen consumed. It is dependent on sex, age, and weight. Weight loss (body fat) often leads to improved VO_2 max.The VO_2 max testing by bicycle assesses three systems: cardiovascular, pulmonary and muscular strength (quadriceps). Any of the three can be the rate-limiting step in the VO_2 max test.

O_2 pulse

O_2 pulse is another way to express your fitness, but it is newer and will require more research to understand the pitfalls. You can ask for it from the person who does your testing. If it is not a part of their standard printout, it can be calculated. O_2 pulse is the amount of oxygen you are consuming per beat of your heart. You will want to know the O_2 consumed at a certain point in time and divide it by your heart rate at that time. You use the maximum heart rate to know your maximum O_2 pulse. Your O_2 pulse should go up in direct proportion to your heart rate elevation

Respiratory exchange ratio (RER)

The respiratory exchange ratio is the ratio of expelled VCO_2/VO_2 consumed. When you exercise, you increase the amount of CO_2 you create because that is the by-product of respiration (one of the ways your cells make energy). When the ratio is $\geq$1.1, the effort is considered optimal for the VO_2 max test. This is the RER that your team will use to assign a target heart rate for HIIT training; when the RER=1.1. If you don't reach an RER=<1.1, you haven't worked hard enough, or you might be sent for further testing to exclude heart or lung problems that would prevent you from achieving a high enough level of work.

If you improve your VO_2 max, you can improve your lifespan.

Physically active people 50–59 years of age had very similar VO_2 max data as those inactive at 20–29 years of age, showing that training programs reduce the rate of expected age-related VO_2 max decline.

> ***Meaning that middle aged people who workout regularly will slow their rate of decline to the extent that they can compete with sedentary youth.***

For every 5 ml/kg/minute reduction in VO_2 max, patients were subject to a 56% higher likelihood of cardiovascular risk factor clustering.

> ***Meaning that if your VO_2 max falls, as you would expect it to as you age, you have a higher risk of heart attacks.***

For every 1 ml/kg/minute increase in VO_2 max, patients were subject to a 15% lower likelihood of death (all cause).

> ***Meaning that if you increase your VO_2 max, you reduce your chance of dying.***

For every 1 MET (3.5 ml O_2/kg/minute) increase in VO_2 max, patients were subject to a 12% improvement in survival.

> ***Meaning that more than one researcher is concluding the same thing. If you improve your VO_2 max, you will probably live longer.***

> ***We stress the importance of VO_2 max as a bellwether of your overall fitness.***

Summary: VO_2 max and Longevity

We directly test the VO_2 max at your first visit, establishing a baseline. With weight loss we expect an improvement in VO_2 max because, in our program, the weight loss is mostly (if not all) fat loss. It is common to see an improved VO_2 max in the first quarter of our program. The improvements often continue for 2–3 years, if training is sound.

While mortality benefits might be seen even with less than the "recommended exercise guidelines," improvements in cardiovascular health come with considerably more effort. This is especially well demonstrated with short-duration HIIT. This is true at all fitness levels, though the least conditioned benefit the most. Naturally, those intensities would need to account for current conditioning, but a progressive HIIT training protocol is likely to yield a much higher benefit to patients than the moderate intensity recommended in many current guidelines.

Like with all training programs, we emphasize the value in establishing a "sweet spot" where your hard efforts are optimally balanced with gains.

In other words, you can expect a degree of good stress and improvement, but you should not be overly stressed. Give it time, the improvements will come with the right training program.

We strive for everyone to find the "sweet spot" where their effort yields the gains they are looking for, without giving up on the program. The changes we hope to help patients make are lifelong changes—not short-term fleeting gains. The most constructive way to approach finding your sweet spot is to make the best choices today that you can make. Separate past choices from today's choices. By approaching your decision making in this way, you are more likely to make, on the whole, more higher quality choices than lower quality ones.

Other tests you might expect from the trainer performing your *needs analysis*

Table 6.1

Tests for Measuring Health-Related Physical Fitness

	Test
Cardiorespiratory Fitness	▪ **Cardiopulmonary exercise testing** ▪ Field tests: step test, 1.5 mile run test, 1.5 mile walk/run test
Body composition	▪ **DXA scan** ▪ Waist circumference ▪ Waist to hip ratio ▪ BMI ▪ Skinfolds
Muscular strength	▪ **One rep max testing** ▪ Grip strength
Flexibility	▪ **Sit and reach** ▪ Modified sit and reach
Balance	▪ **Balance error scoring system (BESS)** ▪ Standing static balance unsupported eyes open ▪ Standing static balance unsupported eyes closed
Muscular Endurance	▪ **15RM testing** ▪ Sit-ups ▪ Curl-ups ▪ Push-ups ▪ YMCA bench press test

Adapted from Medicine ACOS

Training Program Variables Part VII

*N*ext, we will discuss the variables that are selected and manipulated in an exercise-training program. As a program progresses, these variables are varied either singularly or in combination to continue adaptations. At the end of the day, sustainable intensity is what determines gains. Frequency of workouts also plays a role in determining the intensity of your training program. Below is a common formula of the variables that determine the intensity of a single workout session.

Intensity=(Force*Distance*Load)/Rest Periods

Intensity

Intensity is what produces gains.

We dedicate a section entirely to intensity because it is an essential ingredient to progress in training programs. It is also a commonly neglected part of a good training program. The art of a top-notch training program is providing the balance between intensity and sustainability. The *LG sweet spot* describes the balance of gains with effort. At a certain point the gains might not be worth the effort, and might work against your motivation. Finding this balance is a very important part of your communication with your coach or care provider. When eustress, the stress that creates progress in a training program, turns to distress, goals are often delayed or abandoned. Staying in the game is essential to winning it. You are encouraged to keep in mind the irreplaceable value of intensity, but that it can be a double-edged sword. Without intensity, no progress or change will be achieved. The same can be said for too much intensity.

Figure 7.1

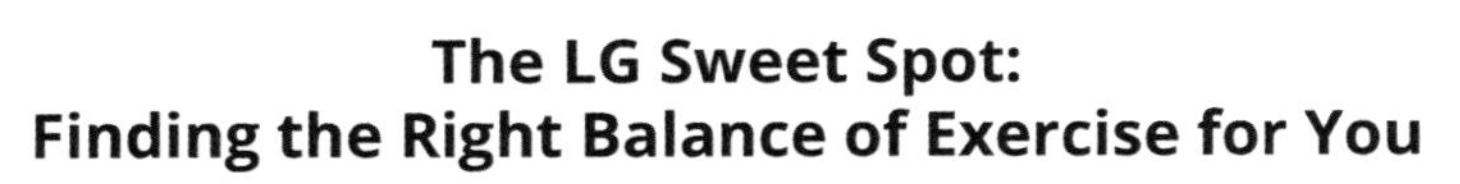

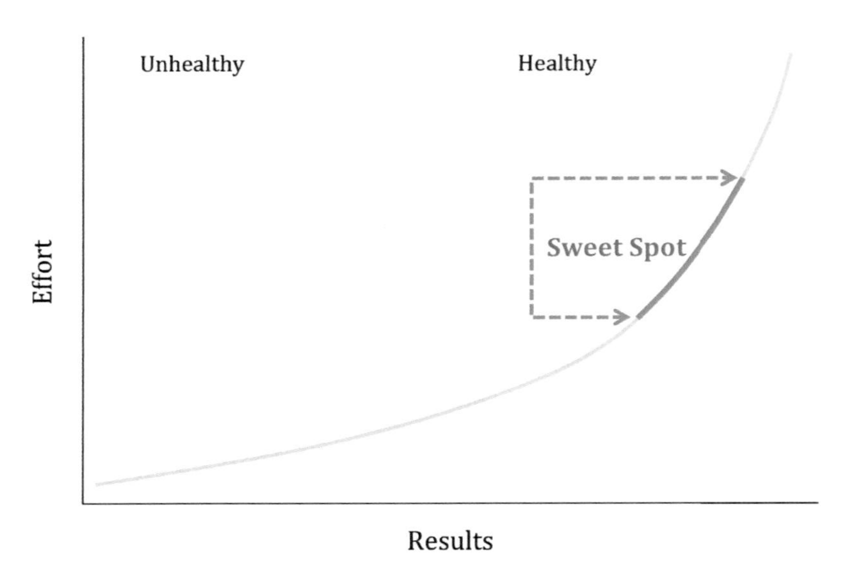

Adapted from Leake

Intensity is correlated directly with duration and the degree of elevation of your heart rate. The more time you spend at an elevated heart rate, the more intense the training. The higher the elevated heart rate, the greater the intensity. When heart rate exceeds the lactate threshold, intensity markedly increases.

> ***Intensity of exercise is closely correlated with body fat loss.***

The harder you work, the more fat you will burn. When you get your heart rate above 90%, your fat burning goes up. The lactate threshold is usually around 90% of the heart rate, thus underscoring the value of achieving or exceeding your lactate threshold. Some will argue "fat burning" mode is at heart rates in the 55%–60% range of your max heart rate. Perhaps that is true if you spend an inordinate amount of time at that pace. Fat burning begins when glycogen stores are gone. Once you achieve lactate threshold, you start to tax the cell, and glycogen stores rapidly diminish.

Below we discuss variables of intensity in resistance training programs. Later, we discuss intensity with respect to aerobic training.

Frequency

The term frequency is the total amount of exercise routines performed throughout the week. The higher the frequency, the higher the volume of training.

Volume

In resistance training, training volume refers to the weight lifted in a single *session*, as opposed to frequency, which refers to training routines throughout the *week*. Volume usually references resistance training but aerobic or HIIT training and be characterized in analogous ways.

For resistance training, the volume of a session is the total weight lifted in that session. Volume can contribute to overall intensity, but does not inherently include the time to perform the volume of weight, and thus by itself, might not reflect intensity.

Total Volume = Weight lifted*Repetitions*Sets

As a general rule, achieving bigger muscles (hypertrophy) requires higher volume. Advanced athletes require higher volumes to achieve training goals and make progress because their muscles have adapted.

In aerobic training, volume refers to the time run/cycled/rowed, or miles run/cycled/rowed during a session.

Load: 1RM and 3RM

In resistance training, the load describes how much weight is being lifted as a percentage of the maximum that you can lift one time (in that exercise). The maximum you can lift in a particular exercise is called the 1RM or the one repetition maximum.

An athlete may determine either a 1RM or 3RM depending on their training level and needs. A beginning weight lifter will probably not be able to determine a true 1RM because it would require adaptations and a better understanding of technique than beginning athletes have. A 3RM is usually sufficient in the first year of resistance training.

A useful formula for estimating 1RM from known maximums of higher repetitions is as follows:

1RM = Weight Lifted*(1+[0.033*n])

** where n is number of repetitions*

A trainer or coach might use a full training session to determine the 1RM of key core exercises, such as squats and chest presses. The extrapolation of the 1RM from these exercises can allow other exercises and their "maximums" to be prescribed. Assistance exercises, which are single-joint, small muscle group exercises, such as a bicep curl, are generally never performed at <5RM.

Various loads can then be prescribed according to periodization for training for a specific sport. Each percentage of the 1RM is roughly correlated to a maximum number of repetitions. The chart below captures the spectrum of repetitions that would be expected according to the percentage of the 1RM being prescribed. An athlete who can maximally lift a load 15 times would expect to be lifting about 65% of their maximum (1RM). For example, if an athlete can squat 100 pounds 15 times, but not 16, it is estimated their maximum squat would be about 150 lb. Although that system is a rough estimate, it is not entirely accurate. The further away the estimate is from the actual load lifted, the less reliable it is. The example above probably underestimates the athlete's 1RM. In part, metabolic systems dominating in hypertrophy are considerably different than those dominating in maximum strength. The most practical and useful way to determine an estimate of an athlete's load schedule is to use their goals and direct maximum repetition accordingly. An athlete whose goal was predominantly power, would want to test as close to 1RM as possible. An athlete whose goal was predominantly hypertrophy would be best served starting the season testing 15RM.

Table 7.1

Scale of 1RM and Training Loads

RM	1	2	3	4	5	6	7	8	9	10	12	15
%RM	100	95	93	90	87	85	83	80	77	75	67	65

Adapted from Baechle et al.

There are a variety of ways to create the progressive overload pattern needed to make gains. Loads can be linearly advanced, meaning they can be advanced in simple stepwise increases. They might also be more undulating or irregular, depending on the athlete's training goals and competition schedule. Submaximal loads are useful in facilitating recovery in an athlete suspected to be near overtraining. The decision to progress the load is constantly re-evaluated by the coach, week to week. As a general rule, the 2+2 pattern might be useful in determining when to increase load. The 2+2 pattern states that if two additional repetitions can be performed on each set in two consecutive workouts, then the load can be increased.

As you can see, in resistance training, load is prescribed as a percentage of your maximum. Thus, it is an indicator of intensity. Though not typically referred to in this way, the aerobic equivalent of load would be the percentage of maximum heart rate, which is our assessment of intensity.

Sets and Repetitions

A set contains repeated bouts of the same exercise. Often times, a set will include 3–5 episodes of the same exercise repeated multiple times. The number of times an exercise is performed in each set is referred to as repetition. Therefore an exercise contains a limited number of sets with a specific number of repetitions. Resistance training goals can be generally categorized as power, strength, hypertrophy, endurance, and speed. Below is a table that provides rough estimates of the loads, sets, and repetitions that facilitate those goals, but keep in mind all elements—power, strength and hypertrophy—are being developed by the exercise. One is being *more* developed than the others according the variations of loads, sets, and repetitions.

Table 7.2

Estimates Of Load, Sets And Repetitions

Goal	Load (% 1RM)	Goal Repetitions	Rest Periods
Power	80–90	1–5	3–5 min
Strength	>85	<6	2 min
Hypertrophy	67–85	6–10	1 min

Adapted from Baechle et al.

Intensity is the key to progress. Managing the positive elements of stress, interspersed with rest, is pivotal to leveraging intensity to benefit.

In resistance training, intensity variables for a single workout session include the total volume of weight lifted and rest periods between. The total volume of weight lifted is a product of load, sets, and repetitions. Frequency is another variable that impacts the overall intensity of a training program. Frequency considers all exercise sessions for the week. A chart below shows the relationship between these variables and intensity in a resistance-training program.

Weight Training Volume = Sets*Reps*Weight

Resistance Exercise

Warm-up, Selection, and Order

Part VIII

Introduction

Training order selection is important to maximize gains and accomplish specific goals. Exercise selection order pertains to a single workout session, like volume.

A workout session typically includes a warm-up period to literally warm up the body. Tissues move more fluidly with higher temperatures. The warm-up period also serves as a signal to the body/mind to prepare for whatever typically follows. For a person performing resistance training, the warm-up is followed by weight lifting. A warm-up should not deplete muscle glycogen stores or contribute to dehydration. A warm-up for a resistance-training program might include a 5-minute light jog to increase the heart rate to not more than 60%–70% of the maximum heart rate.

Exercise order

Faster, more complex, exercises are first

As a general rule, power and more complex exercises are performed first, when the athlete is focused and relatively energized. Exhaustion is a goal of a resistance training session—performing complex intense exercises near exhaustion is ineffective and unsafe. The following order is recommended as a general guideline: Power is performed first, if it is in the spectrum of exercises for that session. Last will be the small muscles performing assistance exercises.

Table 8.1

Basic Principles of the Exercise Session

Principles
Warm-up
Power exercises - I *Structural exercises performed explosively; might be 2-5 reps*
Structural exercises - II *Core with spine loading (Olympic lifts)*
Core exercises - III *Multiple muscles more than 1 joint (compound movement)*
Assistance exercises - last *Single muscle group*
Large muscles before small
Exhaust muscle group before moving to next muscle group
Aerobic or VO_2 max training after resistance training
Stretch last

Adapted from Myers et al.

Varying the exercise routine

1. **Circuit training.** Most commonly used by a beginner. Exercises are performed sequentially, usually on a nautilus-type machine during a structured period. The goal is to move through the circuit; gains in lean mass and aerobic capacity are less than those from more advanced routines.

2. **Pre-exhaustion tactic**. Most commonly used by athletes. Compound movement is used to pre-exhaust a group. Assistance exercises follow the compound movement. For example, the chest press will pre-exhaust the triceps muscle group. After performing the chest press, 2–3 triceps exercises will follow.

3. **Push-Pull tactic**. Most commonly used by advanced athletes. An agonist muscle group exhausted, followed by an antagonist muscle group. The goals of the push-pull routine are the following:

a. Increase intensity and frequency
b. Improve conditioning with shortened rest periods
c. Introduce new exercises to trained muscle groups
d. Emphasize training technique and core stabilization

4. **Three-day split routine** goals:
    a. Increase intensity and load while allowing adequate time for recovery
    b. Increase lean body mass
    c. Emphasize training technique and core stabilization

After a discussion of aerobic exercises, we will discuss the concept of periodization, which places all of the training exercises into a structured schedule to cover a full season (usually 1 year).

Aerobic Training

Part IX

Cardiovascular health is best assessed by VO_2 max testing, as we have discussed. Cardiovascular health decreases with age, with declines of 8% per decade up to the eighth decade, when 20% declines can be expected. Intense exercise directly improves cardiovascular health, reduces or eliminates DMII (with concurrent nutrition changes), and reduces cancer.

Thus, efforts to reduce the rate of decline in cardiovascular health result in reduced mortality and improved quality of life. Sedentary people or beginners (we like to think of as the potential athlete), athletes, and elite athletes all benefit from training programs that improve VO_2 max. The athletes that stand to gain the most are the beginners.

Typical recommendations often are limited to 30–60 minutes a day, 3 times a week. However, the value of HIIT is well established in all levels of athletes. Similar HIIT exercise prescriptions might be applied to the less conditioned; they stand to gain the most. The time demand of HIIT training is considerably less than traditional aerobic training, with as little as 14 minutes 3–4 times week, in two weeks showing significant VO_2 max benefits. In a study comparing HIIT training for 135 minutes (including recovery periods) with those undergoing less intense but longer, training (630 minutes), similar cardiovascular improvements were shown in both groups. Substantially less time (21% of continuous aerobic training) was required in the HIIT training group.

We use something similar to the Coggan Power scale to determine training intensity, and we apply descriptors for ease of communication. Following is a variation of the Coggan Power scale with expected physiological changes for each zone of the scale. Untrained individuals might rate perceived exertion (RPE) higher earlier in training because they are unaccustomed to training.

Table 9.1

Modified Coggan Power Scale

Level	Name	Average Power	Average HR	Description
1	Active Recovery	<55%	<68%	▪ Light spinning, low-intensity exercise, too low to induce significant adaptations. ▪ Minimal sense of effort or fatigue. ▪ Zero concentration to maintain pace. ▪ Uninterrupted conversation is possible. ▪ Active recovery activity during training.
2	Endurance	56–75%	69–83%	▪ Typical long slow distance training. Could do all day. ▪ Low sense of effort or fatigue. ▪ Minimal concentration required at highest end . ▪ Uninterrupted conversation is possible. ▪ Complete recovery might take ~1 day.
3	Tempo	76–90%	84–94%	▪ Low to moderate sense of effort or fatigue. ▪ Requires concentration to avoid slipping to lower levels of intensity ▪ Conversation must be paused periodically. ▪ Complete recovery might take more than 1 day.
4	Lactate Threshold	91–105%	93–98%*	▪ Near threshold training. Beginning levels of HIIT training. ▪ Continuous conversation usually not possible. ▪ Might be episodic due to difficulty in executing. ▪ Consecutive days of training at level 4 possible with proper recovery
5	VO_2 max	106–120%	>100% **	▪ Typical intensity of longer (3–8 min) intervals intended to increase VO_2 max. ▪ HIIT training efforts ▪ High sense of effort or fatigue. Rarely sustainable over 40 minutes. ▪ Continuous conversation not possible. ▪ Uncommonly trained consecutively.
6	Anaerobic Capacity	>121%	-	▪ Sprinting effort, rarely sustainable for more than a few minutes ▪ Heart rate lags effort and intensity. Power meter might be more useful in training. ▪ Severe sense of effort or fatigue. ▪ Conversation impossible. ▪ Consecutive training not typical.
7	Neuro-muscular Power	-	-	▪ Plyometrics ▪ Severe sense of effort or fatigue. ▪ Conversation impossible. ▪ Consecutive training not recommended.

Adapted from Allen & Coggan
**Might not be achieved during initial phases of effort(s)*
***Percentages based on max heart rate and max power.*

Aerobic design variables include prescribing an exercise mode (running vs. cycling for example), a training frequency for the week, the exercise duration for each bout of exercise, and training intensity. Training intensity can be manipulated by effort output (all-out vs. 80% heart rate or VO_2 max), work/rest ratios, and variables specific to the modality, such as running or cycling uphill vs. flats.

Below, we discuss the three major groups of aerobic training; Long slow distance (LSD), high intensity interval training (HIIT) and concurrent training (both).

Long Slow Distance (LSD)

Do it now and then (once a week)

Most data published on the aerobic long slow distance modality is related to elite athletes. Thus, in the aging population, the generalizability warrants deep skeptical consideration.

As a reference, elite athletes train about 15–30 hours per week. In general, they follow a lactate threshold pattern, spending 80% of the time below and 20% above the threshold. For the recreational athlete, there is almost no data. The American College of Sports Medicine (ACSM) guidelines for recreational athletes are below.

Table 9.2

ACSM Guidelines For Cardiovascular Stimuli in Recreational Athletes

Mode/type	Any activity that uses large muscle groups, is maintained continuously, and is rhythmic and aerobic in nature
Frequency	3-5 days/week
Intensity	**40–85% (40–50 % for deconditioned)** of Heart Rate Reserve (HRR), or 64–94% (64–70% for deconditioned) of maximum heart rate
Duration/time	20 to 60 minutes of continuous or intermittent (10 minute bouts) aerobic activity
Progression (rate)	Stage 1: Initial Stage 2: Improvement Stage 3: Maintenance

The recommendations offered by the ACSM are based on heart rate, not lactate threshold, and are prescribed for the beginner athlete. The intended distribution of work can be grouped according to time spent in specific zones. ACSM zones differ from the zones discussed above, but range up to 87% of the heart rate established at VO_2 max. Athletes tend to adjust intensity according the prescribed method for the workout. For example, training intended to be longer and slower tends to become faster and shorter. Thus, even in some athletes, training often fails to reach the prescribed intensity.

Studies show regular runners have about a 50% lower death rate than similarly aged people who don't run.

HIIT (~Anaerobic Aerobic)

The core of your heart program (3–4 times a week)

High-intensity interval training encompasses a broad range of exercises that share the common pattern of rapid and sustained elevation of heart to near maximum, followed by a recovery period of at least 15 bpm, followed by additional cycles of elevated/recovered heart rate. Below is a spectrum exercises that are all HIIT variations with all-out, 40-second sprint interval training (SIT) being the most intense.

It is important to be aware that the literature often confuses HIIT training and high-volume training, and ascribes high-volume training to injuries and risk. For example, top runners might expend up to 7.2 met hours per day (1.5 hours of ~5 met hours running). The safety of such frequent, high-volume work has come into question by recent studies. However, this was one study, and all were post heart attack patients. These are not sprinting runs. By definition it is not possible to truly sprint more than 400 meters at elite levels.

We recommend HIIT training, which is low-volume, but high-intensity because of the degree of energy output during the interval. High-volume and long-duration exercise might lead to intense stress on the body, but it should not be confused with low-volume HIIT training. HIIT training, as we prescribe, is well established in the literature as safe and healthful.

Determining the target heart rate is best with VO_2 max testing. In the absence of VO_2 max testing, the Karvonen method is handy. With increased intensity, type II muscle fibers are recruited for power, promoting conversion to type IIc.

Karvonen Method of Target Heart Rate Determination

Age-Predicted Maximum Heart Rate (APMHR) = 220-age

Heart Rate Reserve (HRR) = APMHR - Resting Heart Rate (RHR)

Target Heart Rate= HRR*Exercise intensity (% of max) + RHR

Figure 9.1

Variety Of HIIT Training Exercises

SIT	Sprint Stair Climbing	Sprint Cycling	Sprint Elliptical	Sprint Rowing	Sprint Swimming	Rapid Repeated Olympic lifts

*** SIT- sprint interval training (running)*

Interval training can be performed in a variety of modes, such as running or cycling, but also at different time intervals. As a general rule, total interval distances for running usually do not exceed 2 miles, as sustained effort beyond this distance usually results in less intensity for the workout.

Training the slow glycolytic metabolism system to process lactic acid more efficiently requires prescriptions of intervals of 1.5–3 minutes. Training the fast glycolytic metabolism system to process lactic acid more efficiently requires prescriptions of intervals of 0.5 to 1.5 minutes. Training the phosphocreatine system to process lactic acid more efficiently requires prescriptions of intervals of <30 seconds. Recovery periods might allow complete recovery or partial recovery. A more complete recovery allows for a more complete repeat interval.

Varying ratios of work to rest can be used to create a progressive interval-training program. To progress, one might extend the length of the high-intensity interval, shorten the recovery interval, or add more intervals. By changing the work to rest ratio to 1:9, the intensity is increased. Thus, a sprinter who takes about 12 seconds for the 100M event might require 2 minutes for a full recovery. Changing the 12 seconds of work/120 recovery to 12 seconds of work/108 seconds of recovery might sound like a small change, but the sprinter will notice it.

There are an infinite number of variations possible in interval training programs. The point of the interval is to allow more work to be done with less fatigue, thus maximizing the benefits. The method used to elevate the heart rate doesn't matter, except that it should be above the lactate threshold. This allows for your preferences to be accommodated in the plan, which means you are more likely to do your workout.

Table 9.3

Benefits of HIIT Training

Benefits
Increases VO_2 max
Increases fat use as energy
Improves hormonal profile (transient cortisol, testostrone, and growth hormone)
Reduces mortality
Reduces body fat

Authors have compared HIIT training to higher-volume, longer-duration but less intense aerobic training programs. The data are mixed. However, many studies show HIIT training produces similar results in VO_2 max as the more time consuming aerobic training programs. Thus, HIIT is easily more efficient at reducing cardiovascular disease when compared to long slow distance training.

Potential mechanism of HIIT training effects on VO_2 max

VO_2 max improvements might occur through various mechanisms with anaerobic HIIT compared with aerobic continuous training. Peripheral changes such as improved skeletal muscle arterial venous oxygen difference might dominate with HIIT training. Continuous aerobic training shows improved cardiac output (CO) through improved stroke volume (SV).

Concurrent Training

Build toward having both aerobic workouts and resistance training in your program

Concurrent training is a term used to described training with both endurance (aerobic) and strength resistance modalities (anaerobic). The spectrum of resistance exercise ranges are shown below:

Figure 9.2

Spectrum of Resistance Exercises

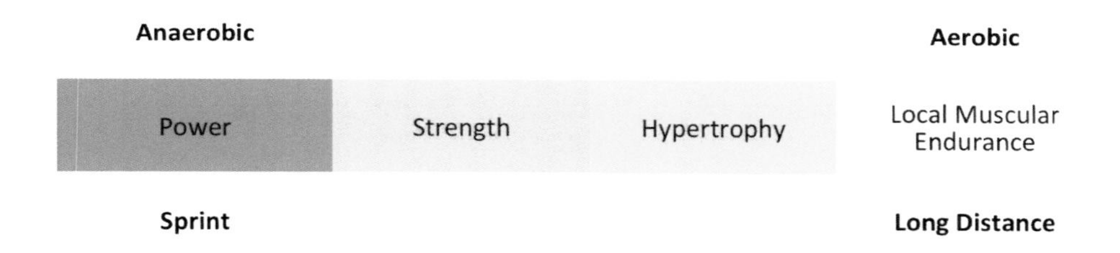

A common misconception among endurance athletes is that anaerobic resistance training will impair their performance, which is largely reflected by the VO_2 max. Not true. A common misconception among strength-focused athletes is that aerobic training will impair their strength. Not true.

The correct concept is that power athletes who rely on very short bursts of force (high velocity strength ≤2 seconds) might see detriments in power with concurrent, long slow distance aerobic training.

> ***The benefit of concurrent training for most aging athletes is that they experience a maintenance or minor improvement in aerobic fitness (VO_2 max) with maintenance of lean mass and substantial increase in body fat reduction compared to either modality alone.***

Overreaching is a term used to describe the thought that combining different exercise modalities results in interference with one or more outcomes of training, such as power, strength, hypertrophy, or VO_2 max. The most accepted theory of overreaching involves programs that result in large amounts of muscle damage. Endurance aerobic training is found to be the primary determinant of the interference effects that result in the clinical setting of overreaching.

Concurrent training can be performed using several modalities, including, among others, running, cycling, stair climbing, rowing, and elliptical training.

It is generally best to perform the aerobic exercise after the resistance exercises if you train both in the same day.

The effects of resistance training are blunted from the effects of aerobic training unless there are 12–24 hours of rest. When the effects of concurrent resistance training in runners are compared with cyclists, runners have a significantly higher probability of reducing strength and hypertrophy. In part, this observation might be explained by the fact that cycling more closely emulates the strength exercises of the lower extremities. In addition, running uses substantially more eccentric muscle action than typical compound movements like squats or cleans. The eccentric muscle action is speculated to result in more muscle damage. For this reason, it is especially important to maintain sufficient protein intake when you train concurrently.

Runners who train concurrently with resistance exercise tend to maintain a higher VO2 max and more substantial fat reduction.

Figure 9.3

Combining a Heart Program with Resistance Training Gives the Best Results

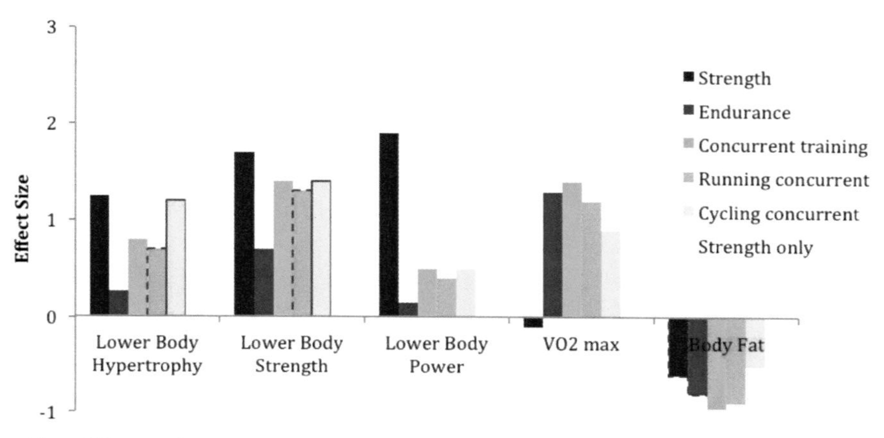

Adapted from Wilson et al.

Skeletal muscle is dynamic, as are bone turnover processes, but faster. Skeletal muscle adapts to loading patterns by metabolically and structurally accommodating the task required. In aerobic endurance athletes, type 1 muscle fibers might selectively hypertrophy but the dominant adaptation is increased protein synthesis (therefore building) in the mitochondrial subfraction. On the other hand, high-intensity resistance training results in type 2 muscle fiber hypertrophy with the dominant adaptation increased protein synthesis of the myofibrillar subfraction. Training, over time, results in more specific adaptations.

Studies suggest resistance training programs should be performed before endurance exercise (or on alternate days) to avoid impaired results.

Overreaching is determined largely by effects caused by endurance training. Those effects are modality and body part specific. Losses in power (~45%) are primarily experienced in the lower extremities when concurrent training programs are combined with lower extremity endurance exercises. Upper extremity power is not significantly affected. Strength, which is essentially slow speed, is not affected by concurrent training. Since power is essentially high velocity speed (< 3 seconds), the factors that affect the rate of force development are likely impaired with concurrent endurance exercise.

> ***When HIIT training was incorporated instead of endurance training, no losses in power were observed in a study assessing collegiate basketball players.***

The remaining benefits of concurrent exercise training were observed, including increased VO_2 max, reduced body fat, increased strength and power relative to either strength resistance training alone or HIIT training alone. Similar benefits as those from HIIT training were seen in collegiate baseball players, which actually showed increases in power, rather than reductions. A theoretical diagram is provided below, showing the potential overlap and competing adaptations with various training programs.

Figure 9.4

HIIT Training Overlaps With Heart Health and Strength Goals

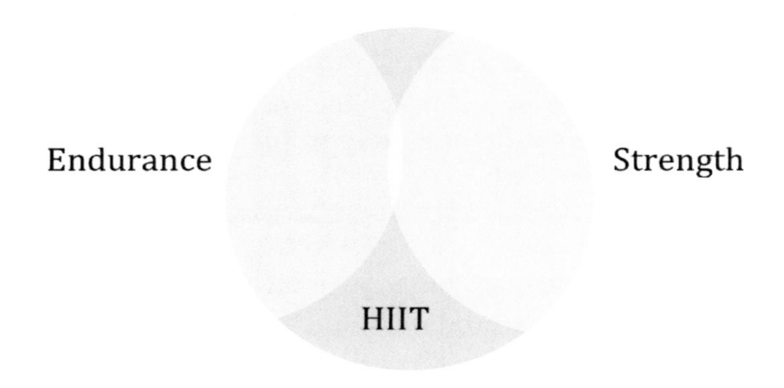

Adapted from Wilson et al.

Summary: Aerobic Training

The well-established benefits of traditional continuous aerobic training are not to be dismissed with the relatively new enthusiasm for HIIT training.

> ***HIIT training can serve as a time-efficient alternative to traditional aerobic training as well as a way to vary an exercise program to encourage adherence and reduce boredom.***

With our patients, we emphasize HIIT training because the parameters are easily transformed into a prescription you can follow. Also, we believe many people are more compliant with time-efficient programs. Higher compliance means higher success rates. Additionally, HIIT training results in substantial body fat reduction but maintenance of lean mass, which complements the goals of aging well.

We do not encourage high-volume, low-intensity endurance training unless that is a specific interest of the patient and if their goals encourage compliance. However, we do recommend periodic (up to once weekly) longer-duration, moderate-intensity endurance training such as a 7K run in a heart rate zone of 3.

We recognize that much more data are required to confirm the long-term benefits with HIIT training compared to traditional continuous aerobic training. Most HIIT studies have been limited to short intervals, such as six-week time periods.

> ***Training intensity is an important variable in creating a progressive program. Too high intensity might result in non-compliance. Too little intensity might have a similar effect.***

Using heart rate (as a reflection of tested VO_2 max) and work/rest ratios are essential. You should use a heart rate monitor each time you work out. A plethora of programs are now available for most smartphones. They will capture heart rate data and for the interested cyclist, power data can be captured as well.

In a well-executed program, you will work toward a concurrent training program that includes, among other modalities, alternating strength resistance and HIIT training with an occasional longer duration aerobic session. You might not start with such a program, but that is the goal.

Program Design — Part X

Where Are You in the Spectrum of Lifetime Athletics?

The first step in assessing your needs is to determine where you are in the spectrum of lifetime athletics. The lifetime process starts with a basic knowledge of how to work out. We call this training literacy. It is a commonly neglected part of new training programs. Our advice is to get a solid foundation in training literacy, even if you think you already have one. The best way to do that is to find a good trainer.

> ***Taking the time to find a good trainer and spending the money until you have that foundation will greatly increase your likelihood of success.***

The system we use to identify where you are on the lifetime training scale is adapted from a Canadian system of promoting lifetime fitness. It includes 7 stages of lifetime participation in fitness that athletes might experience. The first three stages capture the skill set needed to train; they establish training literacy. Stages 4, 5, and 6 are those in which skills are applied to develop a competitive level of training. Competition is encouraged at all age levels, with the most important competition being self-competition. This group of stages promotes the physical, mental, and emotional development of the athlete. The last stage is about developing the skills and executing a prescription of lifetime participation in athletics.

It is not uncommon for patients to feel like they aren't making progress or are failing in their efforts at the gym. In fact, there is a lot of neurological "learning" involved with pushing weights around. It takes your mind time to make those connections. With a good trainer, those connections are made more quickly. Sometimes just by contracting the muscle at the right time during a movement will help your brain make those connections. Beyond how to lift a weight, there are things that you might do inadvertently that work against your goals. For example, if you do your aerobic workout before your resistance training, your body will not respond as favorably to the resistance session. Or, if you do not take sufficient rest, your body won't recover and rebuild. All of these things seem intuitive and deceptively simple, yet it might not be.

You might overestimate your level of training literacy, which can be a real obstacle to progress. It is far better to underestimate your training literacy level and fill in a few gaps you did not know were there, than to jump ahead missing fundamental principles that might take years to fix.

A good trainer will take your personal interests in specific activities and use them to create an effective and useful resistance program. Before you know it, you might be doing activities you never considered, just because you can.

Time availability is commonly a limiting factor for busy people. One of the early steps we suggest is for you to get into a daily routine of doing a structured session. Perhaps one day will be with a trainer, thus a bit stressful, and the next will be Pilates in a group setting. The one indispensable exercise for busy people is low-volume HIIT training. We prescribe it to nearly every patient in our practice. It works. In 18–22 minutes you can be confident you have productively deposited assets into your Heart Bank. How you do your HIIT training is up to you. Sprinting is the most effective way to get the heart rate up, but you can cycle, row, or even climb stairs if you are moving fast enough.

In your training team, look for all of the above elements in their prescription to you. Below, we list 3 tenets we believe you will find in any sound exercise program.

Table 10.1

Tenets of Program Design

Create adaptations Prevent plateaus Avoid boredom

Adapted from Baechle

A good program design is an *effective* program design. It incorporates your level of current fitness, specific interests, time limits, and physical limits. Your goals must be clearly understood and incorporated into the program design. You must perceive a benefit or you will not participate.

Program Design Goals

Identify which tools (processes) you will use to get to where you want to go (outcomes).

The results of a program design are outcomes from specific training stimuli. They are the outcome goals. The program design is the aggregate of the process goals.

As an example, if you want to hike up and ski down a mountain but are only a novice, you know you have to *do* several things to ensure success of your outcome. Those things you identify that you have to *do* are your process goals. Focus on your process goals and the outcomes will materialize.

Process Goals:

Goal 1: You plan to hike a mountain in the summer to assess your cardiovascular fitness.

Goal 2: You plan to take ski lessons to assess your ski skill level.

Goal 3: You plan to improve your cardiovascular fitness.

- a: You plan to start a HIIT program 2xs/week and build to 4xs/week.
- b: You plan to train once a week at altitude for much longer than HIIT training.

Goal 4: You plan to incorporate muscle endurance weight training to improve leg strength.

Goal 5: You plan to learn to use skis to "skin up" the mountain.

Goal 6: You plan to take an avalanche safety course to improve your odds of survival.

Outcome Goal: Climb and ski a mountain.

Each one of the process goals can be broken down further and further until you have a tangible stepwise plan. The goal of your *Needs Analysis* is to establish your outcome goal and the pathway or process goals that will get you there. The program design is the sum of your process goals. Ultimately, your program design will be laid out in a daily schedule. However, you have to start with the big picture first (outcome goals) and work with a knowledgeable team to choose the processes that will be most effective at getting you there.

> ***The better your care provider understands what training stimulus produces what result, the more likely you will perceive successfully working toward your goals.***

You need a knowledgeable team to help you choose the right tools. If the training stimulus does not lead to the outcome you are working toward, then you will perceive the program as a failed program and not participate. An effective program design implements the principles described earlier in the chapter:

The *Needs Analysis* is the key assessment that determines the specific training stimulus implemented to accomplish the goals. The plan is the Program Design.

GAS: General adaptation syndrome 3 stages: Adaptation, Resistance, and Exhaustion.

Progressive: A training program providing clear progressive stress.

Overload: Each training event should create overload.

Overcompensation: The result of healing stronger; requires rest.

SAID: Specific adaptations to imposed demands.

Avoid overtraining—Rest is essential to growth

Exercise selection

Exercise selection is determined by your *Needs Analysis*. Nearly all sports benefit from resistance training, including long distance running. Resistance exercises come in many forms and should be tailored to optimize your specific interests. Exercises can be categorized according to the number of joints involved, whether or not spine loading is a dominant feature, and whether small or large muscle groups are being moved. Categories are described below:

Core exercises are central to an effective resistance-training program. They include multiple joints and large muscles. Examples include the leg press and chest press.

Assistance exercises use 1 muscle group and 1 joint. They can complement core exercises and are often used in rehabilitation. An example is the bicep curl.

Structural exercises are core exercises that load the spine. An example is the squat.

Power exercises are structural exercise that are performed explosively, usually ≤2 seconds. Olympic lifts are power exercise. Examples include the clean, snatch and jerk.

Training frequency

Training frequency is the number of training sessions per week. It includes all of your training episodes—resistance, aerobic, HIIT, stretching, plyometrics etc. Training frequency is an important factor to adjust to minimize overtraining, maximize gains and in competition, to strategically peak at the right part of the season. Aging patients typically require more rest in order to avoid overtraining.

Factors that influence training frequency include the level of fitness, experience level of the athlete, volume and intensity of the sessions, training objectives, time available, and age.

Table 10.2

Factors Influencing Training Frequency

Factors
Level of fitness
Experience level
Volume and intensity of the sessions
Training objectives
Time available
Age (older athletes require more recovery time)

Adapted from Baechle et al.

Periodization

Part XI

*P*eriodization is the process by which a season or seasons of workouts are planned to achieve a specific goal. In the untrained athlete who is rapidly progressing, a periodization program might not be effective until baselines are firmly established. For Olympic athletes, periodization might include a 4-year period. Periodization minimizes plateaus by consistently creating adaptations. It is comprised of micro-cycles (weekly), meso-cycles (a few to several weeks) and macro-cycles (the year). Most athletes are periodized over a one-year period, or 1 macrocycle.

Planned periodization allows management of stresses to optimize gains through intentional adaptation cycles. Training stimuli usually include a varying amount of resistance training and aerobic training. Training stimuli must continue to change to promote adapting and progress. Rest periods are critical elements of periodization, as they allow adaptation to new stresses. Basic principles of developing the periodized program are shown below.

Table 11.1

Basic Principles of Periodization

Principles
Rest period lengths are proportional to exercise intensity
Rest period lengths are proportional to exercise volume
Women require more recovery than men
Elderly require more recovery time than young adults
Larger muscles require more recovery than smaller muscles
Anaerobic action requires more recovery than aerobic action
Sound nutrition and select supplements promote faster recovery
Physical therapy techniques promote faster recovery
Hormone optimization promotes faster recovery

Adapted from Baechle et al.

Just like resistance-training programs, periodization programs can have varying patterns. However, a shared key element is that periodization involves progressive overload.

The pattern of stress and rest might vary to include patterns such as linear or non-linear patterns within a microcycle (week) or mesocycle (months). A non-linear periodization refers to the pattern of high-intensity workout followed by a less intense workout, followed by another high-intensity workout. Periodization is well documented as superior in producing gains when compared with non-periodized programs.

Microcycle

Measured in weeks

The microcycle is a week. It might consist of linear or non-linear periodization. See Table 11.2 for an example of a linear periodization training micro-cycle. The repetitions of non-linear periodization vary considerably, not simply going up each workout. The sets are also nonlinear, to a lesser degree.

Mesocycle

Measured in months

Mesocycles are used throughout the macrocycle (year), and each one is comprised of phases (of one or more microcycles). The phases contain training sessions with a focused short-term goal or gain. Each mesocycle is followed typically by a week of unloading during which workouts are characterized by less volume and intensity. The unloading week promotes recovery.

The typical mesocycles an athlete will train through in an annual competition sport are the pre-season, in-season (competition), post-season (active rest), and off-season mesocycles. Thus, a standard periodized program will usually consist of 4 mesocycles, centered on their sport season.

Pre-season mesocycle

Less resistance training, more sport skills

The pre-season mesocycle is structured for **sport-specific skill development**. As the athlete moves through the in-season mesocycle, the proportion of sport specific-exercises increases, while resistance training peaks. It typically lasts about 14 weeks.

In-season mesocycle

Maintain power focus on sports skills and recovery

The in-season mesocycle is the **competition season.** The focus of the in-season mesocycle is to maintain strength and power gains, sport-specific skills, and rest sufficiently between games to allow peaking again if tournaments are on the horizon. Typically, resistance training volume lessens and sport-specific training increases. It typically lasts 10–24 weeks, depending on the sport and tournament qualifications.

Post-season mesocycle

Recovery period, but not sitting on the couch

The post-season mesocycle is often referred to as **active rest.** The athlete does not have structured workout sessions, but recreational games are encouraged. It is a time for physical and psychological recovery. It typically lasts about 4 weeks.

Off-season mesocycle

Resistance training

The off-season is a testing and conditioning period. The testing is to establish the baseline condition and prescribe a progressive overload series of microcycles. Most hypertrophy and strength/power gains are made during the off-season. Aerobic conditioning testing usually occurs in this period, and according to the sport specifics, will be added to the periodization to maximize conditioning during the in-season.

Table 11.2

Linear Periodization Training Mesocycle

Week	Sets	Repetitions	% 1 RM	Rest (min)	Phase
1-3	3-4	12-15	60-75	1	Hypertrophy
4-8	3-5	8-10	80-85	2	Strength
9-10	4-5	3-5	85-90	3-4	Strength/Power
10-11	3-5	2-4	>90	3-5	Peaking

Adapted from Baechle

Below is a volume/intensity relationship throughout a typical macro cycle. Note the relationship of intensity and competition during the in-season, compared with the off-season.

Figure 11.1

Exercise Volume/Intensity Throughout a Typical Macrocycle

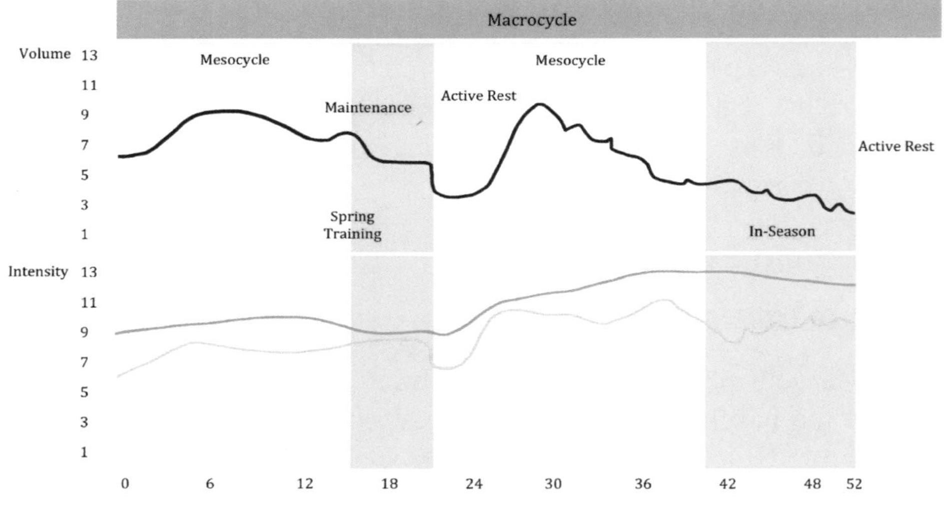

Adapted from Baechle et al.

Common phases of a mesocycle

Hypertrophy phase

First

The goal is to gain mass and prepare for higher-intensity workouts later. Hypertrophy helps the athlete prepare for cardiovascular workouts that will be added later to the periodized program.

Strength phase

Second

The goal is to gain maximum strength. This type of strength differs from power in that it is the maximum achievable for that exercise. The time for achieving a maximum strength effort is usually 3-5 seconds, which is much slower than power.

Strength/Power phase

Third

The goal is to gain maximum power, which is often referred to as high-velocity strength. This phase is considered more intense and will be accompanied by a reduction in volume. Olympic lifts and plyometrics are usually added in this phase.

Summary

In general, each mesocycle has a role in maximizing the athlete's capacity to compete. Understanding the general framework is useful in delivering an effective program for a broad range of patient types:potential athlete, recreational athlete, or elite athlete. The more patients view themselves as lifelong athletes, the more successful they will be. Periodization fills the year with structured and effective phases of maintenance or improvement in physical function. In the noncompetitive aging patient, baseline testing and re-testing is an effective way to emulate the benefits of competition with less stress. More and more products are available that allow for useful data, shared anonymous postings, and comparing of data such that motivated patients do not have to formally compete (and expend resources) to appreciate the benefits of self or anonymous competition.

The important point to note is that everyone can benefit from a program that applies any and all of the training principles to their program. A well-designed program yields better results.

DXA/Screening Tests Part XII

Body Composition

Current status of your body composition

You are already well aware of the expanding, global epidemic of obesity. While data might trickle in regarding improvements on this front, we believe it will be a long, hard battle for several reasons. First, the business of food requires increased costs of food products to maintain equal nutrient value compared with less-handled food. Most food products profit by removing nutrients, adding "filler" ingredients, and marketing to compensate for the lost nutrients and justify the cost.

Second, the human brain is wired to eat when food is available. It requires considerable education and discipline to tone down that innate behavior. Third, food can be, and has been leveraged, to create pleasure. Processed foods in particular capitalize on the overlap in neuronal pathways of pleasure and addiction (to a lesser degree) by providing highly palatable (too palatable), energy-dense, low-nutrient foods. In essence, the processed foods are like an addictive substance, because they stimulate you to eat them but they are not satisfying. More on this topic is provided in the *Nutrition* chapter.

Measuring fat

Nonetheless, the battle for reduced body fat benefits from diagnostic tests, such as dual energy X-Ray absorptiometry (DXA), which accurately measure body fat and is the most accurate and efficient way of measuring body composition in the office setting. With baseline testing, goal setting, and effectively executed plans, periodic DXA scans provide helpful feedback for the patient. Feedback is essential to progress. Since middle age is punctuated with a peak in obesity, it is the optimal time for DXA scanning.

BMI is not accurate or useful for you, though it can be cost-effective for epidemiological studies. It is an indirect and inaccurate assessment of body fat. Specifically, BMI measures the weight divided by the squared height of the patient. It assumes increased weight relative to height is due to body fat. However, many athletes will qualify as overweight or even obese because of the amount of lean muscle relative to their height

For studies whose primary outcomes are body fat, composition or obesity are useful only if they quantify body composition with tools like DXA scanning.

Neither DXA nor BMI are suitable for defining obesity. DXA body fat measurement is not a disease correlate. In the low ranges, BMI can significantly underestimate disease risk. Women are especially likely to be misclassified because of underestimating their obesity-related disease risk. As they age, they become weaker or more frail but not necessarily substantially higher in weight (skinny fat). Thus, the BMI of aging women is less likely to reflect the "normal weight obesity"state. This places those patients at risk for not being treated for evolving metabolic syndrome, insulin resistance, and premature heart disease.

DXA radiation dosage

DXA is a very low dose radiation for exposure. DXA scanning is highly accurate and will provide information about your distribution of body fat as well as bone density information, depending on the protocol used.

The radiation dosage of DXA scanning for bone mineral density is 13 microSieverts for lumbar spine and 9 microSieverts for hip assessment. For body composition assessment, a whole body DXA technique is used, resulting in 42 microSievert exposure.

By comparison, background radiation is estimated at 2400 microSieverts per year; mammography is 400 microSieverts, and adult abdominal computed tomography (CT) is 8000 microSieverts. Thus, the dose of radiation you would receive from a DXA scan is essentially negligible.

Figure 12.1

Body Fat Standards

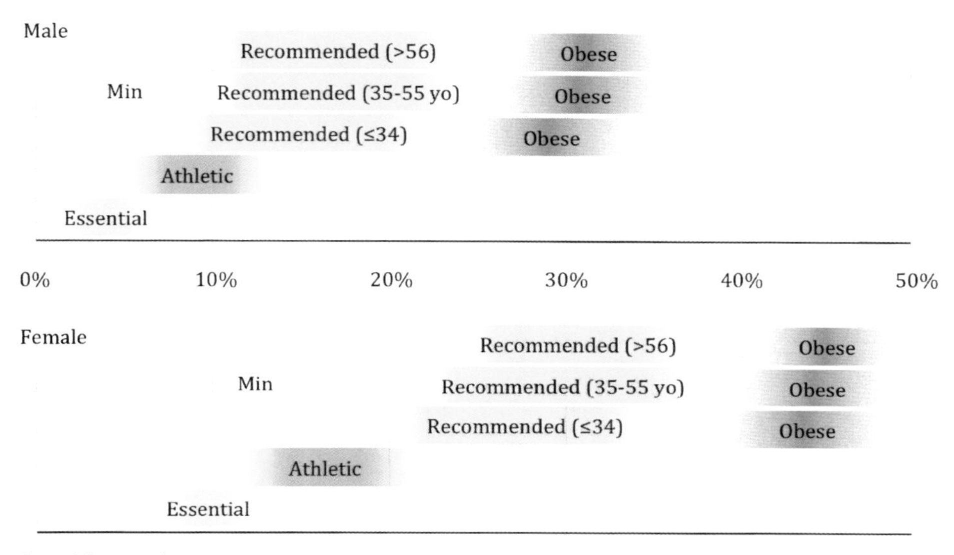

Adapted from Medicine ACOS

Pitfalls and error rates of DXA

Typical errors of measurement of the trunk, leg, and arm lean regions range from 1.3% to 1.7%. Leg measurements are the most consistent measurements. We use 2% as the expected error variation for lean mass measurement with DXA.

For regional fat mass, our typical errors of measurement range from 1.4% to 3.9%. Leg measurements are the most consistent measurements. We use 2.5% as the expected variation for body measurement with DXA.

The myth of the "metabolically healthy obese"

No such condition as "healthy obese"

Reports of "healthy obese" have been popular in the past few years, highlighting the sensationalistic nature of publishing. Similar to studies that have tried to show that omega-3 fatty acids are unhealthy, studies that make the argument a healthy obese population exists are headline-oriented publications. Obesity is undoubtedly unhealthy, though it is likely a result of a metabolic protective mechanism from self-induced toxicity (too many carbohydrates and too many calories). Omega-3 fatty acids are undoubtedly healthy. It might be some obese people are healthier than others, but it is not likely. A BMI of 30 kg/m^2 is unhealthy; at least considering what we know about overstuffed fat cells and their effect on the immune system and oxidative stress from excessive metabolism. Most likely, a study that suggests the possibility of healthy obesity has not studied their population long enough.

Summary: DXA/Screening Tests

Currently, DXA is the most accurate and cost-effective way to assess body fat. The FDA has approved a newly automated method for segmenting fat according to region with DXA. DXA is accurate in distinguishing total body fat, abdominal fat, abdominal subcutaneous fat, and the most harmful fat, visceral abdominal fat.

Prescriptions

Part XIII

*T*he differentiating feature of a good care provider is no longer information or knowledge. Your care provider should understand the obstacles you might experience on your path to health or improvement. Those care providers managing aging patients should focus much more on process goals and less on outcome goals.

This chapter provides the general approach with which we have found success in getting patients onboard with the greatest pill we have to offer, exercise.

Principles of the exercise prescription

Table 13.1

Principles of the Exercise Prescription
Based on Your *Needs Analysis*

Course	Principles
I	Establish the pattern of **exercise**
II	Establish the pattern of **daily** exercise
III	Establish the pattern of **intense** exercise
Last	Establish the pattern of **intense daily** exercise

Adapted from Leake

The beginner athlete

The beginner athlete is any mobile person under 30 BMI. Not everyone is a world-class athlete, just as not everyone is a model or a genius. Focus on making better choices for you more often. Don't worry about what the competition is doing. A successful, sustained training program is about doing what is good for you. Begin with establishing a policy of showing up to the scheduled workout session, then progress to daily workout sessions. Over time, you will build a sense of what you want to push in terms of intensity. Add intensity after you have a well-established routine. Both good and bad habits are hard to break.

We suggest you get your VO_2 max measured first, before your program starts. With a baseline VO_2 max you can measure your progress. It also can be a motivator. And most importantly, if you are not making progress, your team can adjust your program.

> ***You should embrace a sport you like (or liked) for a macrocycle—one year. It can be an entirely new sport or a sport you used to play. By doing so, training has more context than just losing weight, though that might be a sufficient outcome goal.***

With body fat reduction and increased strength, we find even those who do not start the program with a selected sport, often gravitate to one in a year or two. Selecting a sport helps to vary the exercise routine as well, keeping you engaged and working toward your goals. Most importantly, it is fun to be a middle-aged climber, swimmer, skier, or cyclist. Give it a try.

The program below is a program structured for a potential athlete or deconditioned athlete. The most important part of this stage is to get into a routine of daily exercise and begin adaptations in the neuromuscular system that will make more advanced programs satisfying.

Table 13.2

Beginner Athlete Program

Microcycle 1 (Week 1)						
Day I	Day II	Day III	Day IV	Day V	Day VI	Day VII
30 min brisk walking		30 min brisk walking		30 min brisk walking		30 min brisk walking
Microcycle 2 (Week 2)						
30 min brisk walking	30 min brisk walking	30 min brisk walking	30 min brisk walking	30 min brisk walking	30 min brisk walking	30 min brisk walking

Adapted from Leake

Table 13.3

Sample Workout Series A
Total Body Workout

Warm-up	Time 5–10 min	Treadmill Incline 2–5°	Speed 2.8–3.8 mph	Notes
Exercise	2-3 sets	Rest (sec)	RPE	
Chest press	15 to 8	30	8	Do not let elbows go beyond 90°
Wall-ball squat	15 to 8	30	8	Do not let knees pass mid-foot
Seated row	15 to 8	30	8	Maintain erect posture
Hamstring curl	15 to 8	30	8	Lying or seated machine
Overhead press	15 to 8	30	8	Do not let elbows go beyond 90°
Leg press	15 to 8	30	8	Do not let knees pass mid-foot
Lat pull down	15 to 8	30	8	Always perform to the front of the body
One leg floor bridge	N/A	30	8	Hold to fatigue
Plank	N/A	30	8	Hold to fatigue
Finish:	Recumbent	Bike 20 - 30	At Target Heart Rate:	

Adapted from Leake

The Seasoned Athlete

The total body routine is useful in introducing or reintroducing resistance exercise to the major muscle groups without demotivating you.

The routines described below take you, the seasoned athlete, from a basic beginner split routine into more advanced routines, which include plyometrics, yoga, and a specific sport.

Table 13.4

Athlete Program

<table>
<tr><th colspan="9">Progressive Beginner Split</th></tr>
<tr><th>Micro Cycle</th><th>Time</th><th>Day I</th><th>Day II</th><th>Day III</th><th>Day IV</th><th>Day V</th><th>Day VI</th><th>Day VII</th></tr>
<tr><td>1</td><td>AM</td><td>Circuit</td><td>Rest</td><td>LSD</td><td>Rest</td><td>Circuit</td><td>Rest</td><td>LSD</td></tr>
<tr><td>2</td><td>AM</td><td>Circuit</td><td>LSD</td><td>Circuit</td><td>Rest</td><td>C/B</td><td>Circuit</td><td>LSD</td></tr>
<tr><td>3</td><td>AM</td><td>BP</td><td>HIIT</td><td>BP</td><td>Rest</td><td>C/B</td><td>BP</td><td>HIIT</td></tr>
<tr><td>4</td><td>AM</td><td>Circuit</td><td>HIIT</td><td>Circuit</td><td>Rest</td><td>HIIT</td><td>Circuit</td><td>LSD</td></tr>
<tr><td rowspan="2">5</td><td>AM</td><td>Circuit</td><td rowspan="2">Core</td><td>Circuit</td><td rowspan="2">Rest</td><td>TBC</td><td rowspan="2">Balance</td><td>Circuit</td></tr>
<tr><td>PM</td><td>HIIT</td><td>HIIT</td><td>HIIT</td><td>LSD</td></tr>
<tr><td rowspan="2">6</td><td>AM</td><td>2DS</td><td>2DS</td><td rowspan="2">Rest</td><td>2DS</td><td>2DS</td><td rowspan="2">Rest</td><td>2DS</td></tr>
<tr><td>PM</td><td>HIIT</td><td>HIIT</td><td>HIIT</td><td>HIIT</td><td>Yoga</td></tr>
<tr><th colspan="9">Intermediate/Advanced Split</th></tr>
<tr><td rowspan="2">7</td><td>AM</td><td>Chest & Triceps</td><td>Back & Biceps</td><td>Legs & Shoulder</td><td rowspan="2">Rest or Repeat</td><td>Chest & Triceps</td><td>Back & Biceps</td><td>Legs & Shoulder</td></tr>
<tr><td>PM</td><td>HIIT</td><td>HIIT</td><td>Core Flexibility</td><td>HIIT</td><td>LSD</td><td>Core Flexibility</td></tr>
<tr><th colspan="9">Advanced Split</th></tr>
<tr><td rowspan="2">8</td><td>AM</td><td>Chest & Triceps</td><td>Back & Biceps</td><td>Plyometrics</td><td>Shoulder Sprints</td><td>Yoga</td><td>Bag Class</td><td rowspan="2">Rest</td></tr>
<tr><td>PM</td><td>Krav Maga</td><td>Krav Maga</td><td>Krav Maga</td><td>Krav Maga</td><td>Rest</td><td>Krav Maga</td></tr>
</table>

Adapted from Leake

BP: Body Pump; LSD: Long Slow Distance; HIIT: High-Intensity Interval Training; 2DS: 2-Day Split; C/B: Core/Balance.

Microcycle 1–2: Begin with one circuit, advance to two, then three as tolerated. Long slow distance aerobic work 10 to 30 minutes as tolerated. After 6 to 12 weeks, begin interval training and move to split resistance-training schemes.

Microcycle 3: Advance to three days as tolerated. High-intensity intervals 10 to 30 minutes as tolerated. As frequency of sessions increases, interval training can be performed after resistance training.

Microcycle 4-5: Begin with one circuit. Advance to two, then three as tolerated. Long slow distance aerobic work 3 – 5 miles as tolerated. High-intensity interval sessions-25 minutes.

Microcycle 6: Begin with two-day split training. High-intensity intervals 10 to 30 minutes as tolerated. Advance to resistance training 4 days/week. Advance HIIT to 3 days per week.

Microcycle 7: Exercises 2–3 per body part. Sets: 3 per exercise/35 minute total time. Rest intervals 60–90 seconds between sets. HIIT or Core 25 minutes total time.

Microcycle 8: Exercises 2–3 per body part. Sets: 3 per exercise/35 minute total time. Rest intervals 60–90 seconds between sets. Yoga 90 minutes. Bag Class 60 minutes. Krav Maga 75 minutes total time. Sprints 20 minutes.

Table 13.5

Athlete Sample workout Series B

Push/Pull Split Routine

Chest, Shoulders, Triceps, Quads*				
Exercise	2-3 Sets	Rest (sec)	RPE	Notes
Step ups	15 to 10	30	8	Step Up on Bench
Chest press	12 to 6	30	8	Sternum high and shoulders back, 90° in elbows
Leg press	15 to 10	30	8	Maintain proper posture in seated position
Overhead press	15 to 6	30	8	Sternum high and shoulders back, 90° in elbows
Wall-ball squat	15 to 10	30	8	Maintain proper posture, 90° in knees
Dips	12 to 8	30	8	Maintain proper posture, 90° in elbows
Tricep pushdown	12 to 8	30	8	
Back, Biceps, Hamstrings**				
Exercise	2-3 Sets	Rest (sec)	RPE	Notes
Romanian deadlift	12 to 8	30	8	Maintain erect posture during descent phase
Assisted pull up	12 to 10	30	8	Sternum high and shoulders back
Lying hamstring curl	12 to 8	30	8	Maintain proper posture in lying position
Cable row	12 to 10	30	8	Sternum high and shoulders back, maintain erect posture
Seated hamstring curl	12 to 8	30	8	Maintain proper posture in seated position
Bicep curl	12 to 8	30	8	Maintain proper posture, slowly lower weight to full ext.
Hammer curl	12 to 8	30	8	

Adapted from Leake
** Warm-up: Cycle Ergometer 10 minutes; Finish: Cardio and Flexibility*
*** Warm-Up: Cycle Ergometer 10 minutes; Finish: Cardio and Flexibility*

Table 13.6

Athlete Two-Day Split Routine

Day I Full Body		
Exercise	Sets	Rest (sec)
Squat	3	6–10
Barbell bench press	3	6–10
Bent over row	3	6–10
Stiff leg deadlift	2	10–15
Abdominal exercise	3	10–25
Day II Full Body		
Exercise	Sets	Rest (sec)
Deadlift	3	6–10
Seated barbell press behind neck	3	6–10
Close grip bench press	3	6–10
Standing barbell curl (or standing dumbbell curl)	3	6–10
Seated calf raise	2	10–25

Adapted from Leake

Table 13.7

Athlete Three-Day Split Routine

Day I Chest, Shoulders and Triceps *				
Exercise	2-3 Sets	Rest (sec)	RPE	Notes
Flat BB bench press	6 to 10	60	8	Sink shoulder blades down, sternum high, feet planted
Inclined DB chest fly	10 to 12	60	8	Sternum high, slowly descend, forcefully contract
Military press	6 to 10	60	8	Sternum high, slowly descend, forcefully contract
Seated lateral raise	10 to 12	60	8	Maintain posture, raise elbows to shoulder height
Lying BB tricep ext.	10 to 12	60	8	Do not let elbows go beyond 90°
Cable tricep ext.	10 to 12	60	8	Do not let elbows go beyond 90°
Reverse crunches	15 to 25	60	8	Focus on flexion through the hips
Physioball crunches	15 to 25	60	8	Focus on abdominal contraction

Day II Back and Biceps **				
Exercise	2-3 Sets	Rest (sec)	RPE	Notes
Lat pull down	10 to 12	60	8	Shoulder-width grip, sternum high, pull to clavicles
Seated cable row	10 to 12	60	8	Maintain posture - upper body perpendicular to the floor
Single arm row	10 to 12	60	8	Use DB, maintain postural alignment while parallel to floor
Bb shrugs	6 to 12	60	8	Maintain posture, pull shoulders towards ears
Standing bicep curl	8 to 12	60	8	Contract at top of movement, slowly descend
Preacher curl	8 to 12	60	8	Contract at top of movement, slowly descend
Floor extensions	15 to 25	60	8	Lying on stomach w/ arms extended, raise arms and legs
Single floor bridge	15 to 25	60	8	One foot on the ground, opposing foot towards ceiling

Day III Legs***				
Exercise	2-3 Sets	Rest (sec)	RPE	Notes
Walking lunges	10 to 15	60	8	Do not let knees pass mid-foot
Leg press	10 to 15	60	8	Feet shoulder-width, stop at 90 degree knee flexion
Lying leg curl	8 to 12	60	8	Maintain ankle extension through movement
Seated leg curl	8 to 12	60	8	Maintain ankle dorsiflexion
Standing calf raise	15 to 25	60	8	Forcefully contract, slowly descend
Seated calf raise	15 to 25	60	8	Do not let knees pass mid-foot
Planks	Failure	60	8	Go until fatigue

Adapted from Leake
Warm-up: Treadmill 5 - 10 minutes; Finish: Cardio; **Treadmill 5 - 10 minutes; Finish: Cardio; * Bike 5 - 10 minutes; Finish: Stretch*

Aerobic Program Prescriptions

As you know from earlier sections, aerobic training can be generally categorized into LSD or HIIT training. Both increase VO_2 max. In general, an aerobic program design includes the following:

Table 13.8

Aerobic Program Design Variables

Variables
Exercise mode (running, cycling or other)
Training frequency (weekly)
Exercise duration (each session)
Training intensity

Adapted from Leake

Aerobic training intensity is related to the percentage of VO_2 max you are using, which is directly related to your heart rate. Heart rate monitors are becoming nearly ubiquitous and are indispensable for your training. They also add a measure of safety. Please use your heart rate monitor whenever you work out, even doing resistance training. Below is a brief summary list of benefits of either aerobic training program.

Table 13.9

HIIT Is More Efficient Than LSD

LSD* Benefits	HIIT** Benefits
↑ VO_2 max (peak 6–12 months)	↑ Muscle oxidative potential, buffering capacity, glycogen content and time trial performance
↑ Mitochondrial energy production	↑ VO_2 max
↑ Oxidative capacity of skeletal muscle	↑ Levels of cortisol, growth hormone, and testosterone, possibly due to lactate buildup
↑ Lactate clearance	↑ Fat burning due to higher exercise intensity and long-lasting excess post-exercise oxygen consumption (EPOC)
↑ Use of fat, sparing glycogen	

Adapted from Leake

**Intensity up to 70% of VO_2max or 80% maximum heart rate*

***Based upon the concept that the intervals allow more work to be accomplished at higher intensities with the same or less fatigue*

Two variations of the cycle VO_2 max test include the 12-minute run and the 1.5-mile run. Each test is described below.

1.5-mile-run test formula

VO_2 max (ml/kg/min) = 3.5 = 483/time
Time = time to finish 1.5 mile run in nearest 100th of a minute

12-minute walk/run test

VO_2 max (ml/kg/min) = (distance in meters - 504.9)/44.73

Interpreting Your VO2 Max Test

Because the VO_2 max is a strong marker of longevity, establishing a baseline is a cornerstone for any exercise program. Keep in mind that female athletes usually have a lower VO_2 max than their male counterparts. Insist on a VO_2 max or MLSS test before you start your training program. They are relatively inexpensive (~$100) and provide a lot of information your team will need to start you on the right track. Be sure your team gives a full explanation of the results, including anything that might be a red flag, such as failing to meet the minimum heart rate. You will want to ask them about the following values:

Table 13.10

Exercise report	What it means to you
Heart rate when you reach RER=1.0	Beginning of lactate threshold
Heart rate when you reach RER= 1.1	A good target heart rate for your intervals
Maximum heart rate achieved	Training zones are usually based on max HR
O_2 Pulse	Another estimate of training level
Heart Rate Recovery in 1 minute	You will want your heart rate to drop by 12 BPM
Aerobic threshold	The heart rate you do not want to drop beyond between intervals. Usually 0.85

Evidence

Exercise is great for you—the evidence is consistent and powerful

In contrast to nutrition data, exercise data is much easier to validate and apply. It is easier to control parameters of exercise than those of nutrition. However, like all treatments, simply having a prescription will not necessarily result in you being engaged in the therapy. This is true even with prescriptions for pills. Once you fully understand the vast benefits that are already well documented in the literature, the sooner you can start perceiving and experiencing how valuable exercise is to aging well.

Do not be misled by the complacent message in government recommendations. You will need to work for the benefit, but it will come within a month or two of starting a sound program.

There are an overwhelming number of authors who have conclude dthe same thing: that exercise is the greatest pill, ever. For a full list of publications used, see our *Textbook of Age Management Medicine.*

How to estimate caloric intake without counting each calorie

For Men

Your body weight (kg)* 24 hours = Resting Metabolic Rate

For Women

0.9* Your body weight (kg)* 24 hours = Resting Metabolic Rate

Table 13.11

Body Fat Modification

Multiplier	Percent Body Fat (%)	
	Men	Women
1.0	10–14	14–18
0.95	14–20	18–28
0.90	21–28	28–38
0.85	>28	>38

Adapted from Medicine ACOS

Modified resting metabolic rate (MRMR)

MRMR=Resting Metabolic Rate*Multiplier

Total daily caloric expenditure

TDCE=MRMR*Activity Level

Table 13.12

Activity Level Modifier

Multiplier	Activity	Level
1.3	Office, inactive work, studying, sitting	Very light
1.4	Walking, lab, or shop work	Light
1.65	Warehousing, light constructions 1-2 hr	Moderate
1.80	Manual labor, digging, construction, activities like body building, football 2-4 hr/d	Heavy
2.00	≥8 hr of moderate and heavy activities + 2-4 hr/d heavy training	Very heavy

Adapted from Medicine ACOS

Let's work through an example of estimating daily caloric intake

We have a 50-year old man weighing 210 pounds who wants to know how much he can eat each day. Keep in mind, what we print here about calories are still estimates. In the end, how you process each of your meals is still affected by many factors, which we cover in the *Nutrition* chapter. However, it is still valuable to have a rough idea of calorie expenditure.

1. Convert 210 pounds into kilograms: 1 lb = 0.45 kg. Therefore, 210 lb = 95.25 kg
2. Body fat measurements show he has 20% BF (body fat). Modify 95.25 * 0.95 = 90.49 kg
3. MRMR is 90.49 kg
4. MRMR needs to be adjusted based on how active the fellow is. He is a construction worker. Therefore, we take the MRMR and multiply by 1.80 = 90.49*1.8 = 162.88 calories per hour are expended.
5. For a daily count, multiple the final calorie/hr by 24 = 3909 kcal per day.

Most of us do not have very active jobs, so your daily activities will impact how many calories you burn. Keep in mind, as we discuss in the *Nutrition* chapter, your mind/body has a way of driving your appetite to adjust when activity levels change. So exercise is not effective at achieving longer-term fat loss goals because your mind/body will drive you to eat more.

Osteoporosis

Part XIV

Introduction

Prevalence

*O*steoporosis means weak bones. It is a significant health problem, with costs estimated at $22 billion. As the population ages, the incidence of osteoporosis will increase unless efforts are made to prevent it. Treating bones before osteopenia (early bone density loss) occurs will be more effective than waiting for the onset of osteoporosis.

Osteopenia and osteoporosis are measured by bone mineral density (BMD) testing. There is a direct correlation between BMD and the risk of fractures. The increased fracture risk in aging patients is a costly, debilitating risk that can be mitigated by higher BMD, in addition to adequate strength and cognitive function. Exercise early in life is critical to developing a well-supported Bone Bank, as indicated earlier in the chapter. Vitamin D and calcium are critical elements in maintaining bone mineral density, as are other hormones such as estrogens, testosterone, and other factors. The rate of loss of BMD can be lessened and even reversed prior to the stage of osteoporosis.

> ***50-year-old men have a 6% risk of hip fractures and a 16%–25% risk of osteoporotic fractures in their remaining life period. The number of fractures in men is expected to double by 2025.***

The mortality ratio from fractures in men is 3.17 for the proximal femur, 2.38 for the vertebra, 2.22 for other major fractures, and 1.45 for minor fractures. Based on a fracture risk index, even a patient younger than 65 with only osteopenia has an 8.6% risk of fracture of any non-vertebral body, a 0.4% risk of hip fracture, and a 1.2% risk of vertebral body fracture. Testosterone-deficient patients with symptoms in other domains are at risk for osteopenia/osteoporosis.

A total of about 8 million women are affected with osteoporosis, compared with 2 million men.

Developmentally, prepubertal boys and girls have similar BMD. At puberty, both sexes show increased bone formation relative to bone resorption. For young men, the testosterone stimulates increased periosteal bone apposition, and cross sectional diameter accounts for much of the increased BMD. BMD is 5%–10% higher in men compared with women, largely due to the larger diameter of the long bones. BMD peaks around 18–21 years of age.

Beginning around 25–30 years of age, BMD begins to decline at a rate of 0.5%–1.0% per year. The balance of bone resorption begins to exceed bone formation.

The lifetime risk of fracture in men is about 20% by the age of 50

In the elderly, the fracture risk in men rises about a decade later relative to the increase in women. Ethnicity plays a role in fracture risk, with Africans, Asians, and South Americans at lower risk than Caucasian or European people. Men (2 million) are less commonly affected with osteoporosis compared with women (8 million); about 600,000 fractures. However, this figure might be an underestimation. The awareness of preventive therapy (in men) is not nearly as extensive as it is for women. Worldwide, the incidence is approximately 3.5 million fractures in men with approximately 15% of the hip, about 15% in the vertebral body, some 10% in the forearm and the balance distributed throughout the remaining skeletal system. The lower rate of osteoporosis in men relative to women is due to larger bones, less likelihood of falling, and shorter lifespans.

The mortality rate with hip fracture in men is around 2–3 times higher than the mortality rate with hip fracture in women. Thus, it is imperative men's awareness of osteopenia/osteoporosis is increased.

Hormones play a complex role in BMD. Estrogens, testosterone, parathyroid hormone, and "vitamin" D (a hormone) all play important roles in BMD. Studies show that suppression of estrogen, testosterone or vitamin D results in lower BMD.

Estrogen plays an important, if not dominant, role in regulating BMD through bone resorption. Specifically, men with estradiol levels <18 pg/ml have been shown to have a significantly higher risk of fracture. Men with estradiol levels >34.2 pg/ml are relatively protected against fracture risk.

Testosterone's impact on BMD might be less direct. However, in elderly men, lower testosterone levels are associated with a higher risk of low-trauma fractures. In part, testosterone's impact on fracture risk might be mediated through muscle strength or fall risk.

The figure below reflects age-based mortality rates associated with fractures.

Figure 14.1

Men Are More Likely to Die Than Women After a Hip Fracture

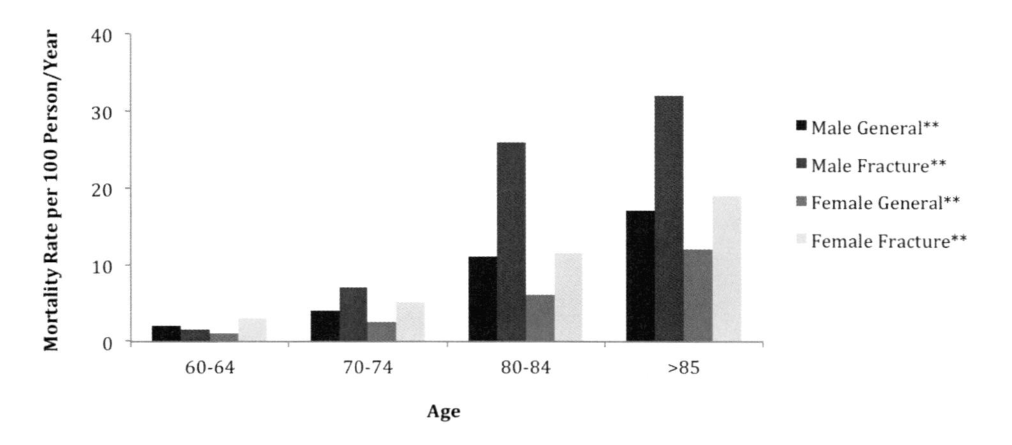

Adapted from Bliuc et al.

***General participants without fractures and fracture patients*

BMD

Bone mineral density measurements are central to the diagnosis of osteoporosis. There are no clinical means to diagnose osteoporosis. Bone mineral content is measured by single and dual x-ray absorptiometry (DXA). The BMD value is derived by dividing the bone mineral content by the surface area from which the content was measured. The accuracy of DXA is >90% in the hip. The presence of osteomalacia (a softening of the bones, often caused by a vitamin D deficiency) might result in an underestimation of BMD. Osteoporotic spurring, sclerosis, or ossification of ligaments might contribute to an overestimation of BMD in the spine and hip. An alternative measuring site includes the femoral neck to exclude the involved joint. Other pitfalls of DXA are listed below.

Table 14.1

Pitfalls of DXA Scanning in the Diagnosis of Osteoporosis

Causes
Osteomalacia, spine/hip osteoarthritis
Soft tissue calcification
Overlying metal objects
Contrast media
History of spine, hip, wrist fracture
Severe scoliosis
Extreme obesity or ascites
Vertebral deformities due to osteoarthritis, Scheuermann's disease
Inadequate reference ranges and operating procedures**

Adapted from Kanis

**calibration, region selection, acquisition mode, positioning; **especially aortic calcification for spine measurements*

Screening and Diagnostic Testing

- Diagnostic testing is performed using DXA. Central DXA focuses on the spine and hips because they carry higher morbidity and mortality when fractured and can predict fracture risk of other bones. Consistent testing, from the same machine, is more likely to produce results that are clinically meaningful. Re-assessment for response to therapy is recommended every 1–2 years.
- Screening testing might include peripheral dual-energy X-ray absorptiometry (pDXA), quantitative ultrasound, and peripheral quantitative computed tomography (pQCT).

> ***T-score is a bone density score relative to a healthy 30-year-old. You want to know your T-Score and keep it above 0.***

Z-scores are age-matched and might understate risk of fracture given the age-related increased prevalence of osteopenia and osteoporosis.

Thresholds of DXA scan values in the diagnosis of osteoporosis

Because the distribution of bone mineral density is approximately Gaussian, regardless of the specific technique to measure BMD, the density values can be scored in terms of standard deviations based on a specific populations, as shown in the following figure.

Figure 14.2

Distribution of BMD in Healthy Young Women

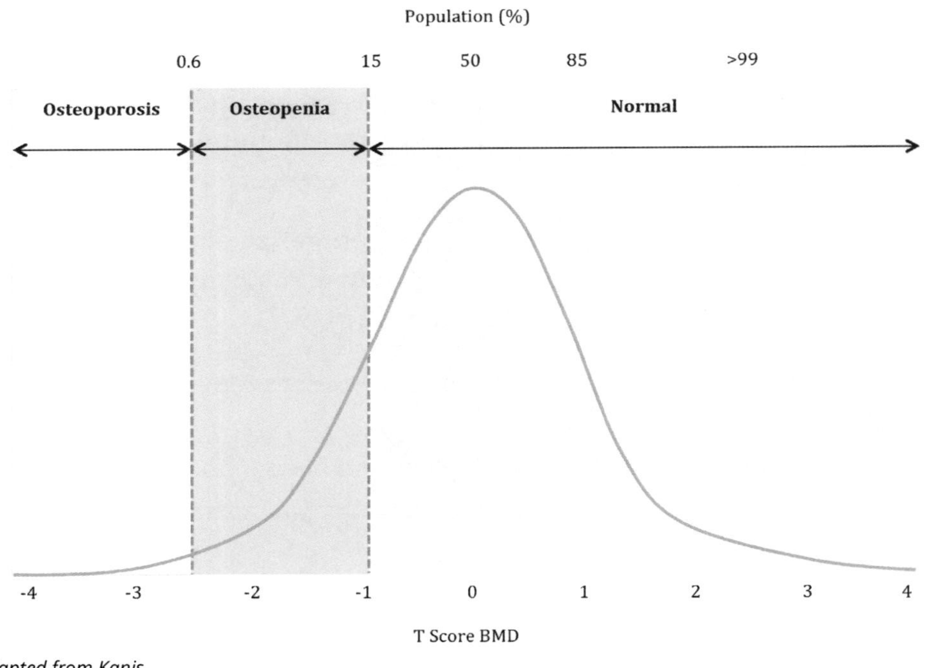

Adapted from Kanis.

A T-score is the number of standard deviations away from the mean for a healthy 30-year-old adult of the same sex and ethnicity as the patient. Below is a short summary of T-score values and their implication for the diagnosis of osteoporosis.

Table 14.2

T-Score Values in the Diagnosis of Osteoporosis

T-Score	Level
≥ -1	Normal
> -2.5 and < -1	Osteopenia
≤ -2.5	Osteoporosis
≤ -2.5 + Fragility Fracture	Severe Osteoporosis

Adapted from Kanis

A Z-score is the number of standard deviations away from the mean for the patient's age, sex, and ethnicity. A Z-score might not be as useful as a T-score because if everyone is osteoporotic, you will get a report that your Z-score is average, which might be falsely reassuring. You will want to know your T score.

Fracture risk

Studies on fracture risk in women are more common than those assessing fracture risk in men. The positive predictive value of osteoporosis (≤ -2.5 SD) for fracture at 50 years of age for the next decade is about 45%.

About 45% of women with osteoporosis at 50 years of age will sustain an osteoporotic fracture in the next 10 years.

However, the sensitivity is low: 96% of fractures in this age group will arise in women without osteoporosis. Therefore, population screening is ineffective.

Fracture risk is correlated with low BMD as well as factors that contribute to fall risk. Fall risk increases with visual impairment, reduced mobility, reduced balance, and higher sedative use. The risk of fracture is 2 times higher for each reduction in standard deviation of BMD (Z-score).

Low BMD is associated with age and low testosterone and low estrogen in both men and women.

Body fat used to be considered "protective" of osteoporosis. Recent studies have clarified previously conflicting data.

As with insulin resistance and heart disease, visceral fat has been implicated in an increased risk of reduced BMD.

Two or more prior vertebral body fractures are associated with a 12-fold increase in future fractures. The incidence of prior fractures increases the risk of vertebral body fractures. Even a few months' use of glucocorticoids increases fracture risk, especially in the vertebral bodies. This risk might be reduced with inhaled preparations or keeping the dose <7.5mg QD. Premature menopause and a history of a fragility fracture are also important risk factors for fractures in aging patients. Hip BMD measurements predict the risk of fracture with more power than vertebral body or forearm BMD measurements.

A more exhaustive list of risk factors for osteoporosis is provided below.

Table 14.3

Risk Factors for Osteoporosis and Increased Fracture Risk

Factors
Ethnicity: White, Hispanic
Age (50–90 years)
Poor physical activity, especially an absence of weight-bearing and resistance training
Poor hormonal bioavailability (including vitamin D, free estrone, calculated bioavailable estradiol, and testosterone, as it supports estradiol production via aromatase
Female sex
Premature menopause
Poor calcium intake/absorption
Primary or secondary amenorrhoea
Primary and secondary hypogonadism
History of fragility fracture
Low BMD
Long-term use of glucocorticoids
Poor visual acuity
Parental history of hip fracture
Neuromuscular disorders
Current tobacco smoking & alcohol intake >2 units daily
Long-term immobilization

Adapted from Kanis

Diagnosing osteoporosis

The diagnosis of osteoporosis is made based on hip measurements, unless there are confounders. The hip fracture is the best predictor of subsequent fractures. Hip fractures also have the most severe complications of osteoporosis fractures, including death.

For men, the cutoff values of BMD are less well defined than for women. However, all conflicting data aside, the few studies that have been performed, overcoming sampling bias, have shown men and women share a similar cutoff value. Thus, a T-score ≤-2.5 SD below the mean defines osteoporosis in both men and women.

Osteoporosis: Impact of Nutrition

BMD begins to decline by age 30. In part, BMD reduction is modulated by both estrogen, and to a lesser extent, testosterone. In postmenopausal women, BMD declines at a higher rate than in men, perhaps due to the more abrupt onset of estrogen reduction. Men typically lag by at least 5–10 years, possibly more, depending on degree of resistance training.

BMD is our best measure for approximating fracture risk, though it is an imperfect approximation due to the inherent errors of DXA scanning, superimposed osteoarthritis, the nature of the T-scoring in general, and also due to the dynamic nature of the skeletal system, with constant turnover and production of bone elements.

Exercise and nutritional elements are important in minimizing osteoporosis. Muscle strength and coordination is likely equally important in preventing fractures. Calcium, vitamin D, vitamin K, appropriate levels of vitamin A, and general diet features of acidity can all impact bone mineral density and thus potentially influence your fracture risk. Exercise can mitigate the dietary pH impact. There are great food sources for all of these, but ask your care provider to be sure you are getting the necessary amounts.

The nutritional requirements to protect against osteoporosis are the same for men and women. The requirements are dietary sources of calcium (1200 mg per day) and sunshine and/or supplemental vitamin D3 to achieve 30 ng/ml serum levels or higher (800-5000 IU/day).

Vitamin D may be given intramuscularly safely in a range of 150,000—30,0000 U, twice a year. Calcium enhances the estrogen effects of reducing bone resorption.

Avoid drinks containing phosphoric acid. Maintaining (or acquiring) a healthy daily intake of vegetables, coupled with sufficient vitamin D3 and calcium intake are the nutritional strategies employed to prevent bone disease.

As you know, omega 3 fatty acids have very positive cardiovascular effects. A few studies have shown data suggesting potentially positive effects on the skeletal system, especially with plant-based PUFAs.

Protein intake drives anabolic activity. High-quality protein is essential to life, throughout life. High-quality protein is most reliably derived from animal sources (wild fish, wild game). As patients age, protein requirements increase. Protein stimulates insulin-like growth factor I (IGF-1), which is known to increase bone-building (osteoblastic) activity as well as calcium absorption.

Data are controversial regarding the net effect of protein intake on BMD. However, considering the range of data, the weight of the evidence suggests dietary protein intake has a mildly beneficial to neutral effect on BMD, and not a negative effect.

Dietary acid/base balance has not been shown to impact BMD significantly.

Osteoporosis: Impact of Exercise

Weight-bearing exercises with a duration of 30-40 minutes per day 4 times a week are recommended to reduce the rate of bone mineral decline. BMD might increase a modest 1%–2%. The earlier in life such exercises are implemented, the better the Bone Bank for the elderly years.

Sprinting will be more effective than jogging, as sprint speed is directly proportional to the energy the runner imparts into the ground. Structural resistance training exercises that emphasize loading the spine are also a powerful tool for increasing bone mineral density. In other words, squats with weights on the bar are useful at building bone strength. They also have been shown to reduce the likelihood of falling.

In elderly people who have already experienced an osteoporosis-related fracture, an emphasis on core strength, lower extremity strength, posture, and balance are valuable preventive measures against future osteoporotic fractures. Whole body oscillatory plates can also be used in immobilized patients.

> ***Exercise might be the most powerful in preventing osteoporosis related fractures by improving mobility, strength, and balance.***

Osteoporosis: Impact of HRT on Women

In women, estrogen therapy is an option for reversing BMD loss. Studies have shown consistent 5%–10% increases in BMD through reduced resorption over 1–3 years with estrogen therapy. More recent studies have assessed low-dose estrogen and found it to be efficacious in dose ranges as low as 0.5 mg (17-β-estradiol oral or 25 μg transdermal). With cessation of HRT, BMD loss resumes at a similar rate as prior to treatment. In about 5 years, the risk is returned to pre-HRT levels.

HRT alone can reduce vertebral body fractures by up to 33%, hip fractures by up to 40%, wrist fractures by up to 40%, and 27% of non-vertebral body fractures as a group.

Menopause is associated with reduced bone mineral density

The vast majority of osteoporosis occurs in postmenopausal women. Some 13% to 18% of white American women age 50 or older have osteoporosis of the hip. Osteoporosis is defined as femoral BMD at least 2.5 SD below the mean of young, healthy, white women of northern European ancestry (i.e., a T-score of -2.5 or below). A T-score between 1 and 2.5 SD below the mean is osteopenia. The prevalence of osteoporosis rises from 4% in women ages 50 to 59 to 52% in women age 80 and older.

Menopause is associated with lower circulating levels of 17-α-estradiol (inhibitory of bone resorption), leading to accelerated bone loss. It should be noted that serum estradiol levels only weakly correlate with rates of bone turnover in postmenopausal women.

Osteoporosis accounts for 90% of all hip and spine fractures in white American women ages 65 to 84. Ironically, most fractures in postmenopausal women are found in women who do not have osteoporosis (similarly, most heart attacks occur in people with normal lipid panels). In the Study of Osteoporotic Fractures, only about 25% of hip fractures and vertebral fractures occur in women with osteoporosis. About 50% of the hip fractures occur in women with at least osteopenia.

For a white American woman at age 50, the lifetime prevalence of any osteoporotic fracture in their remaining life is estimated at 40%. As many as 2/3 of the fractures occur after age 75. The estimated prevalence of hip, vertebral or forearm osteoporosis related fracture is 17.5%, 15.6%, and 16.0%, respectively.

Morbidity and mortality

Table 14.4

Women's Morbidity and Mortality Rates After Osteoporosis-Related Hip Fracture

Facts	Rates
Higher mortality within 1 year of the incident	25%
Require long-term care after a hip fracture	25%
Long-term loss of mobility use	50%

Adapted from Karim et al.

Bone mineral density and fracture risk

In general, after the age of 50, the risk of osteoporotic fracture doubles every 7 or 8 years. The median age for hip fractures is 82 years. The median age for vertebral fractures is likely to be in the 70's.

BMD is a significant determinant of fracture risk in women age 65 and older.

Age is an independent risk factor for fracture, apart from BMD. It would be expected the hip fracture risk would increase 4-fold between ages 55 and 85, based solely on BMD. However, age increases hip fracture risk up to 40 times over the same time span. Thus, aging is a much greater risk to hip fracture than osteoporosis (at least 10-fold greater), highlighting the multifactorial nature of fractures. However, we can do a lot about BMD and very little about aging. As coordination, flexibility and overall fitness diminish, the rate of fractures increases.

Menopause status

Both age and estrogen levels are independently associated with bone loss. Earlier menopause is associated with more substantial bone loss until age 70, when loss levels are essentially equal regardless of age of onset of menopause.

> ***Women lose 2% of their bone density annually beginning at premenopause and extending 3–4 years through menopause. After this period, bone loss diminishes to 1%–1.5% per year.***

Osteoporosis: Impact of HRT on Men

Testosterone therapy's effect on bone mineral density

Testosterone therapy improves BMD of the spine and femoral neck in young hypogonadal men as well as elderly men, in part through increased aromatization (conversion) of testosterone to estradiol.

Improved BMD in response to testosterone therapy is thought to occur, at least in part, through increased available calcium (most studies use 800 mg/QD) and increased calcitriol. In addition, increased aromatization of testosterone to E2 appears to be critical to reducing bone resorption. Estrone might increase by 13% with testosterone therapy.

> ***The data suggest that low estrone and estradiol levels are more significant in predicting reduced BMD than testosterone levels.***

In men, E2 levels are likely modulated, in part, through testosterone, but genomic factors affecting receptor subtypes of estrogen and androgen might also be critical. Regardless of the specific mechanism, men benefit in BMD through testosterone therapy, especially in combination with resistance training and appropriate nutrition.

Sleep — Part XV

Introduction

*S*leep is central to growth and aging. It is probably the domain we know least about with regards to aging. Hopefully, as research continues, it will yield usable diagnostic and therapeutic options for the aging patient. Contrary to what is commonly thought, we do not need less sleep as we age. We simply get less sleep. Below are the sleep stages that we typically experience several times a night.

Sleep stages

Sleep stages are now classified into three phases: wakefulness, non-rapid eye movement (non-REM) sleep and rapid eye movement (REM) sleep.

Wakefulness (W) is comprised of mixed alpha and beta waves and high muscle tone. Usually N1 of REM comes after the W stage, but rarely, N2 or REM might immediately follow if a person is sleep deprived. Beta waves might be intermixed into non-REM and REM sleep.

Non-REM sleep:

- **N1** (1–7 minutes, increasing with age) is characterized by theta waves (relaxed wakefulness), a transitional stage; might have slow rolling eye movements.
- **N2** (20 minutes) is characterized by sleep spindles (sigma waves) and K complexes, and comprises the bulk of sleep (>50%).

- **N3** is characterized by slow-wave sleep or slow delta waves (high amplitude, low frequency waves define this stage). It is the most restorative stage of sleep and diminishes with age. Nightmares and sleepwalking characteristically occur during this stage. This stage has the highest arousal threshold. Patients who awaken during this stage might be confused or disoriented.
- **REM** sleep (active sleep) involves theta wave dreaming (phasic phase of REM, or PREM) and low muscle tone (tonic phase of REM or TREM). Sleep apnea might be most pronounced in this stage. Nightmares might occur in this stage as well as in N3.

Sleep duration is optimal between 7–8 hours per night. It is a common misconception that we need less sleep as we age. We often just get less sleep. In fact, we continue to have optimal health at 7–8 hours of sleep. Sleep duration, in excess or in shortage, results in increased morbidity and mortality. Thus, sleep duration has a U-shaped curve in relation to morbidity and mortality.

Sleep duration variation (short and long) is a known risk factor for cardiovascular disease and inflammatory diseases. A recent prospective study conducted in the Netherlands suggests sleep duration-related increases in cardiovascular disease might be more significant than previously thought.

Those patients with sleep duration ≤6 hours had a higher risk of CVD incidence, and when that is compounded by lower sleep quality, the risk increases further.

Table 15.1

Risks of CVD Incidence According to Sleep Duration

	Sleep Duration, h	Short Sleep HR	Long Sleep HR
CVD incidence risk	≤6	1.15 *(1.63 w/lower sleep quality)*	-
CVD incidence/death risk	≤5	1.48	1.38
Stroke risks		1.15	1.65

Adapted from Grandner et al.

Sleep and inflammation: The common link

Too much and too little sleep lead to more inflammation. Aim for 7.5 hours per night.

Inflammation is a well-established underlying cause of heart disease. To review, the accumulation of LDL cholesterol in a previously damaged artery results in an inflammatory response that can lead to plaque formation.

Obstructive sleep apnea (OSA)

Prevalence

OSA refers to a condition of pauses in breathing during sleep, usually due to an obstruction such as excess fat in the throat area. These pauses can be from seconds to minutes long and can occur up to 30 times per hour during sleep, causing serious drops in oxygen and increases in carbon dioxide in the blood. Sleep apnea is an epidemic largely affecting the obese. Sleep apnea prevalence in the US ranges from 2%–24%, but it is likely closer to the upper margin of this range, considering that many patients are undiagnosed.

Sleep apnea is moderately associated with increased age up to 65 years, body mass index (BMI), neck circumference >43 cm (17 in), hypertension, Chinese and African American ethnicities, and sex (men 2-3:1 compared to women).

OSA is strongly associated with hypogonadism, DMII, obesity (BMI >35), metabolic syndrome, congestive heart failure, atrial fibrillation, nocturnal dysrhythmias, stroke, and treatment-refractory hypertension.

The drive for sleep is closely tied to the level of brain activity during wakefulness, balanced by the circadian alerting system. *Brain activity increases adenosine, which is thought to promote sleep drive.* With sleep, adenosine levels diminish. The circadian alert system serves as a counterbalance to the drive to sleep.

Why some people awaken early

When the circadian system reduces its signaling, the sleep drive dominates, create a strong urge to sleep. During the afternoon, there is a lull in the circadian alert system, allowing for potential sleep drive dominance for an hour or two. This phenomenon, often falsely attributed to big lunches, is the basis for cultural variations of siestas. During the first half of sleep, about 4 hours, the sleep drive easily dominates. After about 4 hours, the circadian alert system might begin to dominate, resulting in early awakenings. When the circadian alert system is desynchronized from the sleep drive, obtaining quality sleep can become very challenging. The desynchronization is the basis of jet lag and shift work-related low sleep quality.

Role of weight loss in treating obstructive sleep apnea

In a randomized controlled study of 264 patients with DMII with an average BMI of 36 and average apnea/hypopnea index (AHI) of 23.2, those who lost 10 kg or more in a 1-year period showed improvements in AHI scores by 9.7. They were 3 times as likely to have complete remission of OSA. The reduction in AHI scores was directly related to the degree of reduction in weight. Thus, in many cases, OSA might be considered simply a complication of obesity in DMII.

Summary: Sleep

Our initial evaluation includes an assessment for risk factors of OSA and patient education on lifestyle modifications to reduce such risk factors. If required, we recommend a home screening test for quality of sleep, potentially followed by a split night sleep study.

Sleep cycles tend to last 90–110 minutes and range from 4–6 per night. Later sleep cycles tend to have longer REM periods. Poor sleep hygiene (late-night blue light stimulation, late night alcohol intake, late night food intake) contributes to impaired first and second sleep cycles, which are critical to GH secretion (and thus to the success of your exercise program).

Early in life, naps or multiphasic sleep dominates, especially in infants. Later, monophasic sleep patterns dominate until people are elderly, when a reversion to multiphasic sleep patterns is often seen. Short-term consequences of sleep deprivation include lower attention, memory concentration, and quality of life.

Long-term consequences of sleep deprivation include increased morbidity and mortality, increased obesity, increased type 2 diabetes, increased CVD, and an increased incidence of depression.

Conclusion

Part XVI

*E*xercise is a crucial element to health. Humans are wired to move, to burn energy, and to use their muscles. Contemporary life has removed the expected physical work from daily life. It must be re-incorporated into people's lives if they are to be healthy. The choices are to return to physical labor or incorporate deliberate, goal-oriented physical activity programs into people's lives. While physical labor might be rewarding, it is not likely sustainable by most people throughout their expected lifetime.

> ***Even those who are intuitive enough to incorporate physical labor into their lives will likely need to shift to a structured training program at some point as they age.***

Training is a lifetime process. Each person is unique and requires an **individual** ***Needs Analysis*** to create an effective training program. It begins with learning how to train effectively with proper technique. Once one's exercise technique is consistent and correct, volume and intensity can be added to accomplish personal goals. Everyone has a different composition of muscle fiber types, metabolic tendencies and capacities, baseline VO_2 max, and response to training. Goal setting must be personalized, as there is no one best way to train for all. There is a best way to train for each patient. Helping you find that path is our goal. Part of our guidance to you on your journey is helping you to make better choices for yourself, daily.

Figure 16.1

Shifting Your Health Choices Toward The Ideal

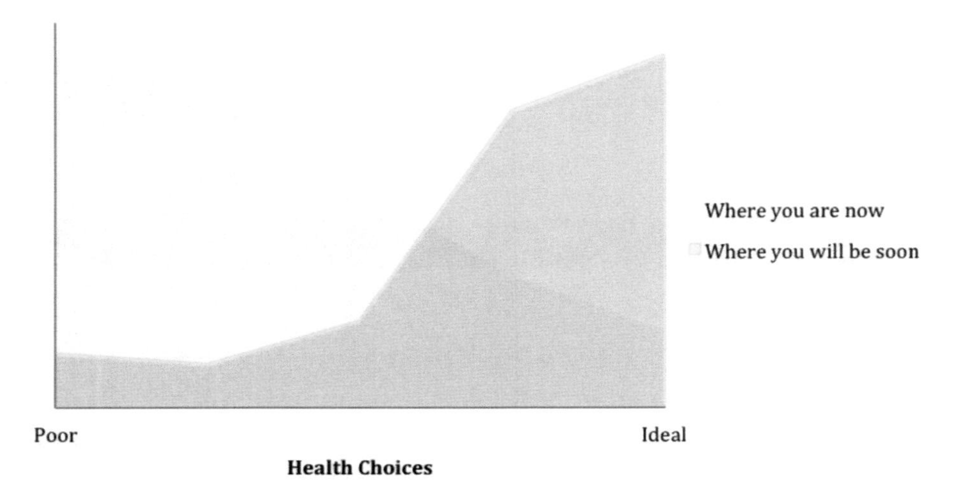

Adapted from Delavier

Each "better' choice is an irrevocable investment. The "better" choice cannot be erased by a less than optimal choice. Strategic concepts are provided below:

Table 16.1

Unlinking Each New Decision from the Last Decision

Make a healthy choice (nutrition or exercise), because *it is an irrevocable contribution to one's health that can never be taken away.*
Don't expect perfection, it will lead to a sense of failure, which leads to frustration.
Frustration leads to the abandonment of the program.
Think what you can do better **today.**
Every decision is done in isolation of the others…it is a new opportunity.
If you failed to make a positive choice, you will have another opportunity soon again.
By **unlinking the decisions,** *you will never be worse than "zero for one."*

Adapted from Leake

When you have a program designed for you, it is critical you are part of designing it. **The best-designed program that you cannot or will not execute is a useless program.** We find that helping you focus on the core principles of fitness without being distracted by sideline issues is essential. Below are the core elements to focus on when you execute your program.

Figure 16.2

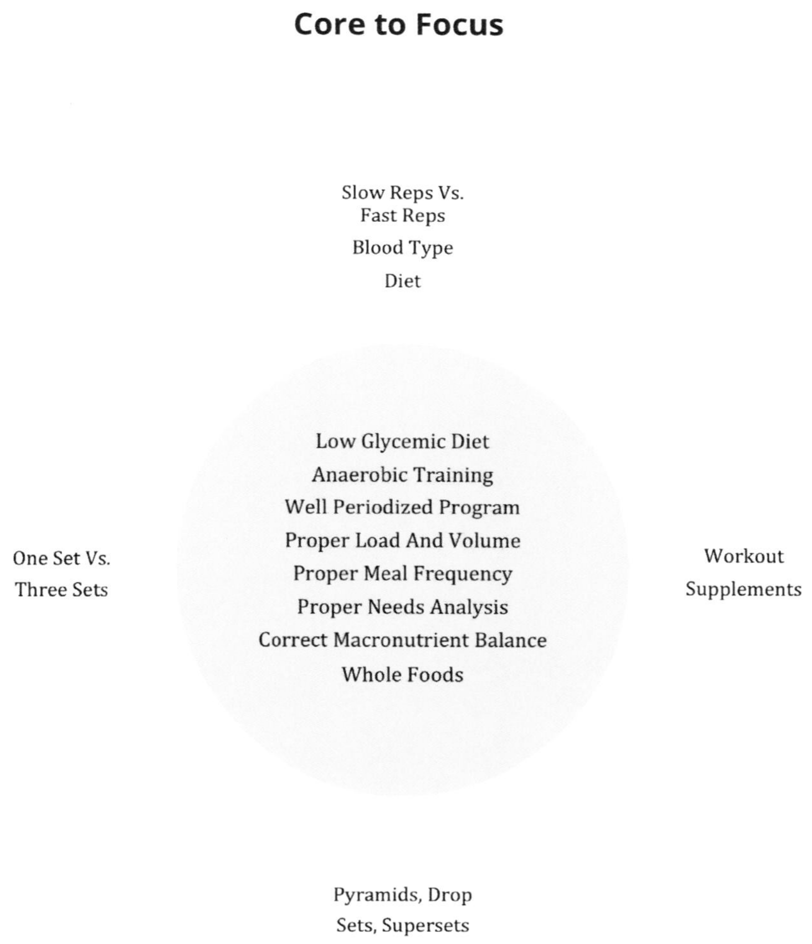

Core to Focus

Slow Reps Vs.
Fast Reps
Blood Type
Diet

One Set Vs.
Three Sets

Low Glycemic Diet
Anaerobic Training
Well Periodized Program
Proper Load And Volume
Proper Meal Frequency
Proper Needs Analysis
Correct Macronutrient Balance
Whole Foods

Workout
Supplements

Pyramids, Drop
Sets, Supersets

Adapted from Leake

It is useful for you to be aware of some of the most common misconceptions in exercise that can be obstacles to your success.

Table 16.2

Biggest Errors in Thinking About Exercise

When you think you can exercise yourself to being thin.
When you overemphasize **exercise duration** at the expense of **exercise intensity**
When you train **aerobically** instead of **anaerobically**

Adapted from Leake

Our approach to exercise prescriptions is shown below:

Figure 16.3

Our Approach to Exercise Prescriptions

I. Establish pattern of **exercise first**	Ii. Establish pattern of **daily** exercise	III. Establish pattern of intense exercise	IV. Establish pattern of **intense daily exercise**

Adapted from Leake

We emphasize that your journey is a lifelong process. There is no need to rush, but we do emphasize consistency. Dedicating a time each day for fitness is crucial to your health. Starting with short but daily exercise routines will be more effective than overextending one day and collapsing the next. When increased intensity becomes part of your training program, days off do become essential to progress. In some training programs, an hour of stretching or Pilates may be used as a lighter training day to facilitate recovery while still keep the momentum of daily involvement. Effective trainers are essential to progress at virtually all levels of training.

Keep in mind that sex differences might impact your results as well. Men tend to be leaner than women. However, women burn more intramuscular fat than men.

Sleep and recovery are essential components of any fitness program. Quality sleep requires more deliberate effort with age. It is a myth that you need less sleep as you get older. Most studies show that optimal health in the aging patient comes with 7–7.5 hours of sleep per night. Several simple guidelines might improve sleep quality dramatically. Such guidelines include the following:

- A consistent bedtime between 9-11 PM
- Cool, dark, and quiet room without blue light (e.g., laptops, iPads)
- Little food and zero alcohol in the 2 hours preceding bedtime
- A non-stimulating bedtime routine is often helpful, such as preparing foods, clothes, and other things for the next day to make mornings more organized.

Throughout the journey, at some point you will likely find a balance between the results you are striving to achieve and the effort you want to put forward to achieve them. It is a wonderful place for you to be able to choose to go the extra mile, or not. Helping you find your sweet spot is a big part of what we aim to achieve.

Ten Top Tips for finding your exercise sweet spot

1. Find a good trainer to help you create an effective program.
2. Wear your heart rate monitor each time you work out.
3. Exercise is not your primary tool for weight loss.
4. Lift weights, it will help you stay out of nursing homes.
5. Work on balance exercises 30–60 seconds a day.
6. Long slow distance is less efficient than HIIT, but good for the heart.
7. As little as 80 minutes of HIIT per week improves length of life.
8. Quality rest is an important part of a training program.
9. Make better choices more often, not perfect choices all the time.
10. It's a journey, not a race. Slow deliberate progress brings success.

CHAPTER III

TESTOSTERONE DEFICIENCY

"If a man does his best, what else is there?"

General George S. Patton

Introduction to HRT — Part I

*L*ife expectancy and, to a lesser extent, quality of life (QOL) have increased dramatically over the past century, fueled by our expanding knowledge of healthy living. Until recently, our lifespan was closely related to the length of the hormone-rich reproductive years.

The past century was an exceptional period in human history, when life expectancy at birth increased from 47.3 years to 78.1 years. In 1900, only 4% of the US population was over 65 years of age. Current estimates by the Centers for Disease Control and Prevention (CDC) suggest that by 2030 19.6% of the US population will be over 65 years of age, with roughly 10% over 85 years of age. The elderly population continues to increase, but men still die earlier than women. Many of these men are testosterone-deficient. Currently, 41% of the US elderly population is male, a statistic projected to increase to 44% by 2030.

Today, our lifespan includes a hormone-rich period followed by a nearly equal or longer period of relative hormone-deficiency.

For women, the transition from an estrogen-rich state to estrogen-depletion is relatively abrupt. For men, the transition from a testosterone-rich state to testosterone depletion is more gradual.

Menopause has always been considered unavoidable, and during the past decade hormone supplementation was believed to be unsafe. Today, estrogen replacement is recommended for most healthy female patients, as detailed in the chapter on *Hormone Replacement Therapy for Women*.

Rigorous population studies have demonstrated that women who took estrogen supplements from the onset of menopause have at least a 20% lower mortality rate, with even lower rates for women who take estrogen supplements for longer periods.

> ***Similar to HRT for women, recent studies of men have shown that testosterone supplementation decreases mortality (from all causes) from 20.7% to 10.3%, a decrease of around 50%.***

Table 1.1

Testosterone Exposure	Person-Years	Deaths	Mortality per 100 Person-Years
Untreated	2290	131	**5.73**
Treated	1190	41	**3.44**

Figure 1.1

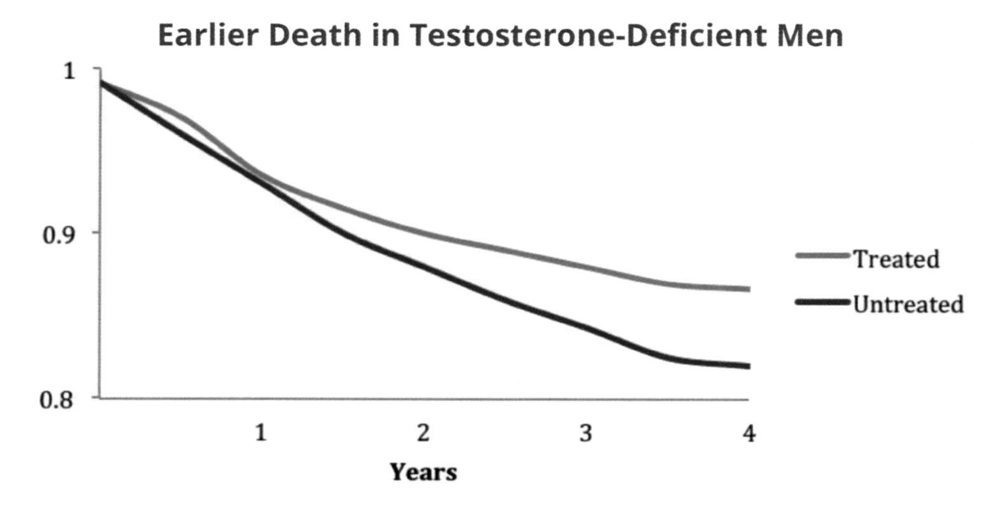

Adapted from Shores et al.

Figure 1.2

Higher Quality of Life with Hormone Replacement Therapy

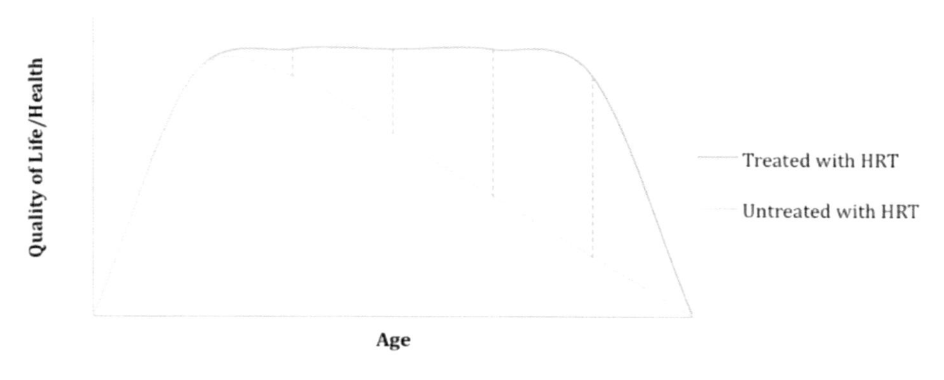

Adapted from Marin et al.

In a perfect world, free of confounding factors such as cost constraints and incomplete data sets, double-blind randomized controlled studies would shed light on cause and effect relationships. *In the absence of such ideal conditions, we instead turn to common sense, the combined clinical experience, and well-designed population studies that show strong correlational data supporting both a longer lifespan and improved QOL with the use of hormone supplementation.*

Fractures and potentially fatal falls were once thought to be the inevitable consequences of old age. We now know that the underlying process leading to osteoporosis begins as early as 30 years of age.

> ***By eating well and engaging in progressive resistance exercises, young men and women can protect themselves from decline by building their Bone Bank and Muscle Bank.***

The reserves in these "banks" can be drawn upon over time. Although bone mineral density (BMD) and muscle strength will still decline, they will do so at a reduced rate, lessening the prevalence of patients at high risk for osteoporotic fractures and sarcopenia (weakness that often leads to disability and the need for assisted living).

As with estrogen deficiency in menopause, the barriers to diagnosing and treating testosterone deficiency will be overcome. This could also dramatically reduce the cost of comorbidity states associated with testosterone deficiency. Building physical reserves to reduce the rate of osteoporosis and sarcopenia will be instrumental in reducing the disability resulting from frailty.

> ***Correcting testosterone deficiency and engaging in an effective nutrition and exercise program not only reduces morbidity and mortality in aging men, but also improves their quality of life.***

As we have learned from our study of women and HRT, there is an ideal treatment window. We believe this is true for men as well. Earlier diagnosis and initiation of hormone-optimizing treatment will provide better results than waiting. As with women, there could be a risk of heart disease associated with starting too late. Men over 35 years of age are encouraged to start educating themselves about testosterone deficiency so that if symptoms arise, they can at least consider the possibility of having this disease. Although the transition for men is not as abrupt as it is for women, the deficiency is no less damaging, and the transition provides a bit more challenge in determining when to start the therapy.

Why Consider Hormone Replacement Therapy?

Longer and healthier life

Testosterone deficiency leads to shorter life spans, lower QOL and increased costs due to an increased incidence of diseases such as obesity, diabetes, frailty and disability.

Total testosterone levels decline at a rate of approximately 1.6% per year. Free and bioavailable testosterone decline more rapidly at a rate of 2%–3% annually. A corresponding increase in sex hormone-binding globulin (SHBG) levels also occurs with aging (approximately 1.6% per year). Among other factors, increased SHBG levels reduce bioavailable testosterone.

Low testosterone levels unequivocally lead to higher abdominal (visceral) body fat, decreased muscle strength, lower BMD and reduced exercise effectiveness, which in turn lead to increased heart (cardiovascular) disease, frailty and disability. The strongest association is likely to be between low testosterone and increased visceral body fat, which is in turn linked to insulin resistance, increased aromatization of testosterone to estrogen, and premature heart disease.

Between the ages of 20 and 80, total testosterone levels decline by 35%; more importantly, free testosterone levels decline by 50%.

Monitoring serum levels of free and total testosterone is the only laboratory measurement available to determine the body's response to exogenous testosterone. However, there is evidence of distinct local tissue environments (or milieus) that are not measurable. These local milieus (in the muscle, fat tissue and other tissues) can have a substantial impact on the net effect of exogenous inputs. For example, muscle-specific insulin-like growth factor (IGF-muscle), which has a strong effect on cell and tissue growth, is produced only locally and is stimulated by circulating testosterone. IGF-muscle is not significantly present in circulating blood. Measuring your testosterone levels is therefore important, but it is only a small window into your overall androgenic environment.

Additionally, the androgen receptor's sensitivity to testosterone and dihydrotestosterone (DHT) affects the overall impact of testosterone on the cell and tissue. Androgen receptor sensitivity decreases with the variation (polymorphism) of the cysteine-adenine-guanine (CAG) repeat length found in exon 1 of the androgen receptor gene.

There are also financial advantages to remedying testosterone deficiency. The cost of treating diseases associated with this condition is extremely high. Reducing these expenditures, by even a fraction, would result in substantial savings. Over a 20-year period, testosterone deficiency might have been directly responsible for approximately $190–$525 billion (inflation-adjusted) in US health care spending.

Table 1.2

US Health Care Expenditures Affected by Testosterone Deficiency

Frailty/Disability	$397.8 billion
Cardiovascular disease	$312.6 billion
Diabetes, including type II	$245 billion
Metabolic syndrome, obesity	$147 billion
Osteoporosis in men, fractures	$22 billion
Total	~$1.1 trillion

In the upcoming chapters, we will discuss the prevalence of testosterone deficiency, the most common diseases associated with the condition, and who stands to benefit the most from testosterone therapy. After establishing the widespread impact of testosterone deficiency on aging men, we present the current data on the efficacy of testosterone therapy and the areas of concern for safety.

Prevalence

Part II

Current data indicate that for each decade of life, the prevalence of testosterone deficiency increases by 17% after the third decade of life.

Introduction

The prevalence of testosterone deficiency has been studied by a number of leading medical societies and panels in the US and Europe over the past 3 decades. The reported prevalence of testosterone deficiency ranges from 2.1% to 39% in studies of men aged 40 and over. The wide range in the reported prevalence underscores the lack of consensus in what defines testosterone deficiency, a topic discussed more fully later in the chapter.

What is the profile of the testosterone-deficient population? Age and body mass index (BMI) are both directly correlated to testosterone deficiency rates. An increase of BMI by 4–5 kg/m^2 is likewise associated with an increased prevalence of 17% every 10 years. Chronic disease states are associated with higher rates of testosterone deficiency. Testosterone deficiency can be masked in smokers, who tend to have increased testosterone levels due to smoking.

Figure 2.1

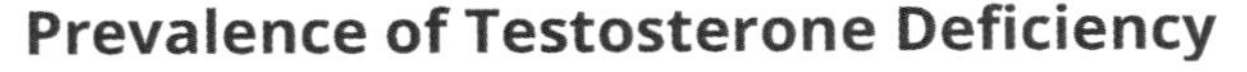

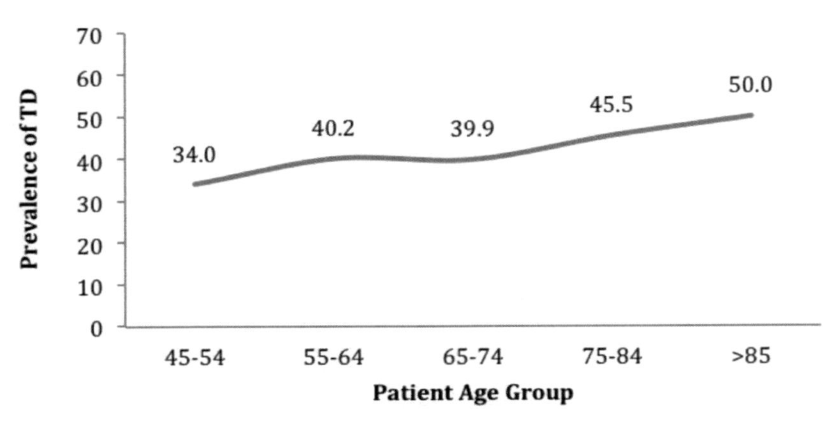

Adapted from Mulligan et al.

Challenges With Current Measures of Testosterone

In addition to the various technical limitations involved in measuring total testosterone and free testosterone in the lab, we should also consider the daily intrapatient variations in testosterone levels according to health status, age, fasting state, sleep, and other factors. Up to 35% of men with low testosterone levels have normal levels within 24 hours, and up to 15% of young men have testosterone levels below the normal range. The significance of low normal testosterone levels in symptomatic middle-aged men is not fully known, but they could be an undertreated patient population. Studies have suggested that such patients are at risk for overall increased mortality (up to 40%); if they are diabetic, they are at increased risk of heart attacks. The measurement of free testosterone (FT) and total testosterone (TT) levels is necessary for managing patients with symptoms of low testosterone levels, but reference ranges should be used as guidelines, not as absolute inclusion or exclusion criteria for the diagnosis of testosterone deficiency.

Individual hormone levels vary considerably from the normal reference range for the entire population. What might be normal for one person might be low in another. For example, if a person who has always had high testosterone levels experiences a 50% drop in their levels, their levels might still lie within the normal range. However, they are experiencing considerably lower testosterone levels than they have in the past. Conversely, a person who has always had levels at the lower end of normal that have not changed in the past 5 years might not experience any new signs or symptoms of testosterone deficiency. We know that the phenomenon of hot flashes in women is a consequence of estrogen withdrawal, not just low estrogen levels. Similarly, men are likely to have symptoms related to testosterone withdrawal, rather than to just low testosterone levels. Those symptoms would not be experienced by the man in the provided example who consistently had low testosterone levels for the past 5 years. The man who experiences a drop from high to low normal levels might be much more symptomatic. Both men still fall within the "normal" population range. Therefore, the signs and symptoms you experience are equally or more important than lab values, particularly if you do not have lab test results from your mid-twenties for comparison. Furthermore, the upper limits of normal testosterone levels in relatively healthy patients with low heart disease risk might provide substantial health benefits, as can be seen in our discussion of the benefits of testosterone.

Resistance to Diagnosing Testosterone Deficiency

Resistance toward diagnosing testosterone deficiency is due largely to a lack of awareness.

The rate of diagnosed testosterone deficiency has risen, yet a number of survey-based studies strongly suggest that testosterone deficiency is undertreated in the aging male population. The Endocrine Society (2009) reported that patients often visited multiple care providers before receiving the diagnosis. Thirty-six percent of men had consulted 2 physicians, and up to 9% had visited 4 care providers before undergoing treatment for testosterone deficiency, which indicates a resistance toward diagnosing the condition.

Up to 35% of patients who reported symptoms of testosterone deficiency did not undergo treatment. Another survey indicated that only 12.2% of men who met the symptom criteria for testosterone deficiency were actually undergoing treatment. Thus, in addition to the challenges involved in accurately identifying the condition's prevalence, there could be several other factors contributing to the resistance in diagnosing testosterone deficiency.

Table 2.1

Why is There Resistance to Diagnosing Testosterone Deficiency?

Why is There Resistance to Diagnosing Testosterone Deficiency?
A mindset that sex hormone deficiency is natural and therefore requires no correction (philosophical perspective)
Lack of screening tests for patients (research perspective)
Lack of consensus on biochemical and clinical criteria (research perspective)
Lack of patient awareness of testosterone deficiency symptoms (patient perspective)
Lack of index for suspected diagnosis (clinician perspective)
Lack of confidence in the available diagnostic tests (clinician perspective)
Lack of knowledge of the correct way to treat testosterone deficiency (clinician perspective)

Biochemical diagnostic criteria are likely to become more individualized and could include information on other androgens, genetic data regarding receptor status (CAG repeat length) and ratios in comparison with other hormones (cortisol, estradiol [E2]) and/or binding globulins (SHBG and corticosteroid-binding globulin).

Studies suggest that additional biochemical markers might also be important for assessing testosterone deficiency and response to therapy.

Is Testosterone Deficiency on the Rise?

Figure 2.2

Testosterone Levels in Men Are Decreasing
More Today Than 50 Years Ago

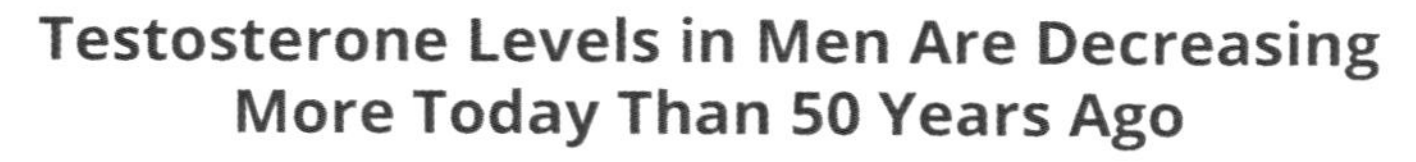

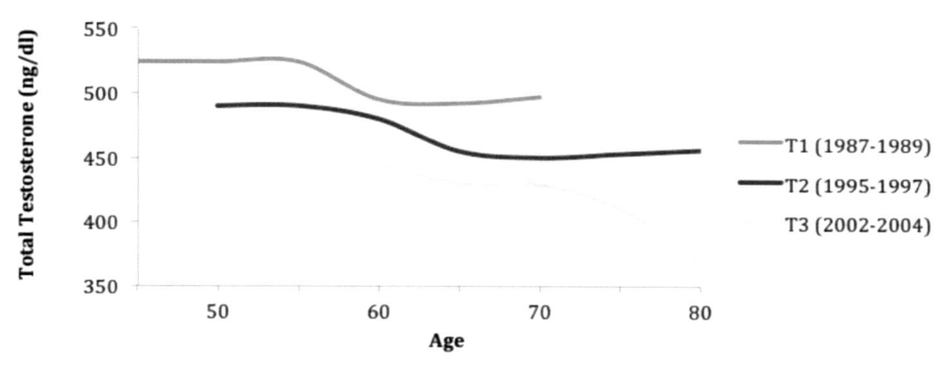

**Crude mean total testosterone concentrations from the Massachusetts Male Aging Study (MMAS) wave (T1, T2, and T3). Estimates are obtained from a generalized additive model with a low smoothing term.*

Screening for Testosterone Deficiency

At present, there are no general screening protocols recommended for testosterone deficiency. The decision to implement testosterone therapy, as with estrogen therapy for menopause, will be prompted by physiological changes observed during the clinical visit. A high index of suspicion for testosterone deficiency by the care provider is instrumental for initiating a diagnostic workup for testosterone deficiency, especially if the symptoms overlap with other disorders such as depression.Finding a care provider with a sound understanding of testosterone deficiency is essential when considering solutions to related symptoms. If the physician does not consider testosterone deficiency in their diagnostic options, the opportunity to undergo treatment for the condition could be missed. In short, find a care provider who is up to date on the literature.

Clinical symptoms of testosterone deficiency can be divided among the physical, sexual, and emotional domains. The emotional domain encompasses conditions related to mood and cognitive performance.

Estrogen in Men

Estrogen is an enigma in men. Our knowledge of how this hormone affects men is very limited compared with what we know about its role in women. In men, increased testosterone levels lead to increased estrogen levels through direct production in the testes and aromatase conversion. The intracellular conversion of testosterone to estrogen is not currently measurable but could have a considerable impact on how estrogen influences certain conditions in men, particularly in terms of bone resorption and blood vessel health.

Estrogen can drop to low levels in men, resulting in paradoxical symptoms such as weight gain, low libido, and bone loss.

Estrogen can also reach excessively high levels in men, leading to symptoms such as breast tissue growth and increased nipple sensitivity. Care providers can prescribe medications that address high estradiol levels, such as aromatase inhibitors (Arimidex/Anastrozole); however, these drugs can have certain adverse effects.

Summary: Prevalence

The rise in testosterone deficiency observed over the past 3 decades is probably attributable, in part, to the corresponding increase in obesity and environmental toxins, such as phthalates found in plastics.

The prevalence of testosterone deficiency in the general male population (as conventionally defined) is about 39%, although the rate can vary depending on the testosterone levels used to reach the diagnosis and the emphasis a clinician places on the symptoms. We do know that the prevalence of testosterone deficiency increases with age and that the prevalence is also influenced by the level of awareness patients and clinicians bring to the visit. If neither the patient nor the clinician considers testosterone deficiency, the condition will not receive treatment. Complaints in the physical, sexual and emotional domains might be attributed to causes other than testosterone deficiency if this deficiency is not considered.

Who Benefits from HRT? Part III

Elderly men are less responsive to testosterone therapy and might be at risk for increased heart disease. The increased likelihood of multiple disorders as we age probably plays a role in this trend. The length and severity of the deficiency is also known to play a role in men's response to testosterone therapy, which further emphasizes the importance of dealing with this issue earlier in life. Blood vessel health also plays an important role in the efficacy and safety of testosterone therapy, which highlights the value of seeking early treatment. Age has an inverse relationship to the effectiveness of testosterone therapy and is an indicator (but not the cause) of ineffective testosterone therapy.

> ***In short, the earlier the treatment for testosterone deficiency is begun, the more likely an effective response is achieved.***

Although they have not been as thoroughly studied as elderly patients, middle-aged patients are logically much better candidates for intervention with testosterone replacement and sound nutrition and exercise programs. One explanation for better results in this population is simply that the supportive local environment, which cannot be measured but know is important (androgen receptors, estrogen receptors, protein synthesis, inflammatory state, endothelial condition), is more sensitive and better maintained in the middle-aged than in the elderly. Furthermore, testosterone therapy complements sound nutrition and exercise programs, further augmenting preventive effects on frailty and potentially dementia.

Testosterone levels decline insidiously, in contrast to the decline of estrogen levels in women. It is therefore harder for men to reach a diagnosis based solely on laboratory cutoff values. The new onset of testosterone deficiency-like symptoms (discussed in the following sections) after the age of 35 should prompt a full evaluation of testosterone deficiency.

Diagnostic Criteria for Hormone Deficiency

Part IV

Introduction

A combination of laboratory measurements and certain signs/symptoms enable the diagnosis of testosterone deficiency. Clinical symptoms prompt the need for laboratory investigation, but laboratory results and symptoms are needed to reach a diagnosis.

The full impact of testosterone on the body is a product of numerous factors, including the total and free testosterone levels measured in the blood.

Testosterone's most interesting actions occur at the cellular and tissue level; effects that can be measured in the laboratory but not in the clinic. These factors can be said to act at a local level and include the androgen receptor (AR), which allows testosterone to bind to it, starting a cascade of action that results in the cell production of other proteins and hormones. This receptor can be very sensitive to testosterone and create numerous proteins and hormones. Alternatively, it can also be very insensitive. The receptor can be found in various forms (polymorphisms), a number of which are known to be associated with various conditions such as baldness and benign prostatic hypertrophy (enlarged prostate). A polymorphism is a small mutation that can result in a significant difference. At the local level, other hormones that affect health and strength can be created, such as IGF specific to muscle tissue. However, it can go undetected in the blood. Testosterone can also be converted into estrogen and DHT at the local level.

FT constitutes only 1%–2% of all circulating testosterone. TT is a combination of FT, tightly bound testosterone, and loosely bound testosterone. Tightly bound testosterone is similar to the "cholesterol on the minibus" discussed in the *Nutrition* chapter. Cholesterol and sex hormones are carried by proteins in the blood. However, the proteins that carry cholesterol are significantly different from those that carry sex hormones, and therefore the names of the "minibuses" are different. The protein that carries cholesterol is known as a lipoprotein, and the protein that carries testosterone is usually SHBG. Loosely bound testosterone is often near albumin, another protein in the blood. However, in this case, testosterone does not completely "board the bus," as it does with SHBG, but rather connects to the side much like a skateboarder hanging onto the minibus door. In this case, we refer to the testosterone as loosely bound to albumin. Thus, testosterone can be found free or bound (loosely or closely). The sum of these testosterone units is what is measured as TT.

In short, testosterone levels can be measured, but the measurement alone does not report the level of testosterone deficiency in an individual. Given that we cannot measure all local effects, we have to rely heavily on the symptoms to reach the diagnosis. Lab studies are important but are mostly a reference point for treatment response rather than the only method for reaching a diagnosis.

Biochemical Diagnosis of Testosterone Deficiency

Forms and measurement of testosterone

Your care provider will typically perform one or two serum assessments of your TT and FT levels. The most important assessments are those of morning testosterone levels, when no food has been eaten for approximately 8–12 hours before the blood draw. Your care provider might ask for a redraw for confirmation due to the wide variation in levels that can occur. Other samples typically drawn at that time include those for other hormones, such as estrogen, and for measuring pituitary function. If your pituitary gland is not functioning properly, it could be due to a testosterone deficiency. AR polymorphisms, although not currently tested routinely, can also lead to reduced testosterone effectiveness. You can ask your care provider whether they test for increased CAG repeat lengths, which are associated with reduced AR sensitivity. For the interested reader, a detailed discussion on this topic, including diagrams, can be found in our *Textbook of Age Management Medicine*.

Clinical Diagnosis of Testosterone Deficiency

As discussed earlier, the three major domains of symptoms related to low testosterone levels include the physical, sexual, and emotional domains. In aging men, determining the effect of low testosterone levels on symptoms is often complicated by co-existing medical problems such as obesity, depression, alcoholism, and chronic obstructive pulmonary disease. Questionnaires can be useful, and some care providers administer the Androgen Deficiency in the Aging Male (ADAM) questionnaire. Our practice prefers a modified version that is more comprehensive.

Table 4.1

ADAM Questionnaire

1. Do you have a decrease in libido (sex drive)?	Yes /No
2. Do you have a lack of energy?	Yes /No
3. Do you have a decrease in strength and/or endurance?	Yes /No
4. Have you lost height?	Yes /No
5. Have you noticed a decreased "enjoyment of life"?	Yes /No
6. Are you sad and/or grumpy?	Yes /No
7. Are your erections less strong?	Yes /No
8. Have you noticed a recent deterioration in your ability to play sports?	Yes /No
9. Are you falling asleep after dinner?	Yes /No
10. Has there been a recent deterioration in your work performance?	Yes /No

Table 4.2 below summarizes the published guidelines for establishing clinical diagnostic criteria for testosterone deficiency. The signs and symptoms marked in bold are considered more common in testosterone deficiency.

Table 4.2

The Three Major Domains of Testosterone Deficiency Signs and Symptoms

Physical Domain	Sexual Domain	Emotional Domain
Muscle ▪ **Decreased strength** ▪ Decreased lean body mass *Bone* ▪ **Decreased bone mineral density*** ▪ Osteoporosis ▪ Mild bone loss* *Fat* ▪ **Increased body fat,* especially visceral** ▪ Decreased insulin sensitivity ▪ Reduced cholesterol processing efficiency ▪ Presence of metabolic syndrome components* ▪ Hot flushes *Other* ▪ Loss of muscle mass ▪ Fatigue ▪ Pre-frailty or frailty* ▪ Low blood hematocrit (blood thickness)	▪ **Reduced libido***[1] ▪ Erectile dysfunction ▪ Decreased/absent morning (spontaneous) erection ▪ Reduced intensity of orgasm ▪ Low sperm levels ▪ Very small or shrinking testes ▪ Breast discomfort ▪ Loss of pubic and axillary hair, reduced need for shaving	▪ **Decreased energy*** ▪ **Depressive mood*** ▪ Ornery/cantankerous disposition* ▪ Decreased overall drive* ▪ Decreased sense of well-being* ▪ Decreased concentration* ▪ Sleep disturbance ▪ Cognitive decline

**The most common signs and symptoms*

Testosterone deficiency is underdiagnosed due to a number of barriers. Chief among these are the absence of clear criteria on signs, symptoms and effective response tests, as well as a lack of awareness.

> ***Sexual symptoms are typically the most specific indicators of testosterone deficiency.***

Physical domain symptoms are very common but are usually dismissed as the expected natural consequences of aging. Emotional domain symptoms are less consistently specific among patients with testosterone deficiency but can also be underreported due to the lack of patient awareness and validated clinical testing.

Weakness (sarcopenia) and bone loss (osteopenia) should also be considered diagnostic criteria for testosterone deficiency. These conditions are best treated before a patient progresses to frailty and osteoporosis. Loss of BMD is known to progress at an annual rate of 1%–2%/year. Weakness, based on the measurement of lower extremity muscle strength, has an estimated annual progression rate of 3%–4% and can lead to disability and loss of independence.

Incorporating additional measures and markers of health status, such as variations in CAG repeat lengths, hormonal affinity to binding globulins, and insulin sensitivity could be of clinical use, enabling a more individualized approach to therapy.

Summary: Diagnostic Criteria

The diagnosis of testosterone deficiency relies on laboratory measurements of testosterone (total and free), as well as clinical signs and symptoms that can be improved with testosterone therapy. Other laboratory studies that could be of value include a search for multisystem hormonal deficiencies. Genetic tests to determine CAG repeat lengths could gain importance in the future as we unravel the impact of the AR polymorphism on androgen action.

Clinical complaints related to testosterone deficiency are of equal or greater priority in making the diagnosis. It is almost universally accepted that clinical signs and symptoms must exist in conjunction with biochemical criteria. Awareness is steadily improving, but patients need to demand that their care providers have a better understanding of testosterone deficiency.

How Can You Benefit from Testosterone Therapy?

Part V

Introduction

*T*he benefits and efficacy of testosterone therapy vary significantly, a reflection of the complex interplay of numerous hormones and hormone receptors, as well as the patient-specific conditions affected by diseases, age, and genetic tendencies. Most of the effects of testosterone therapy are evident within 3 months, especially when combined with sound nutrition and exercise programs. Changes in BMD can take 12–36 months to occur and are heavily influenced by nutrition and exercise.

In the absence of proper nutrition and exercise, the efficacy of testosterone therapy is likely to be limited or negligible, except in cases of erectile dysfunction (ED) and reduced libido caused by testosterone deficiency.

Simply taking testosterone without engaging in a proper exercise and nutritional program is not likely to result in substantial benefits, visceral fat reduction or increased musculoskeletal health. When you combine hormone replacement therapy (HRT) with a sound nutritional and exercise program, the benefits are synergistic.

Muscle strength

Definite benefit

Data from several randomized controlled studies and a meta-analysis suggest that muscle strength will very likely increase with testosterone therapy in both elderly and middle-aged/younger men, as well as in men who are eugonadal (normal functioning testes) or hypogonadal (testes that produce insufficient testosterone). Although this is not unexpected, the fact that many of the studies did not monitor exercise (or did so unevenly) was surprising. Studies on compliance (i.e., how well patients adhere to a program) show that the significant variation in weight loss and muscle strength gain has more to do with the patients' adherence to the program. Exercise is a requirement for depositing in the Bone Bank and Muscle Bank; excessive exercise, however, is not. The same applies to the Heart Bank gains, which are dramatically improved by workouts that challenge the heart, as was discussed in the Exercise chapter.

Muscle strength gains begin at 12 weeks and begin to plateau at 12 months. The gains can extend further depending on training, nutrition, and health status.

Bone mineral density

Definite benefit

Data from several randomized controlled studies and a meta-analysis suggest that BMD will very likely increase with testosterone therapy in middle-aged/younger men; however, elderly men are less likely to see this increase. Men who are eugonadal and hypogonadal could also benefit.

Changes in BMD are probably more closely related to how testosterone is metabolized than to its direct effects. Estradiol, free estradiol, and bioavailable estradiol levels, in addition to the free estrogen index and IGF-1 have been shown to be more closely associated with BMD changes, as detailed in the section on osteoporosis.

Changes in BMD begin at 3–6 months and start to plateau at 36 months. The changes can extend past that point depending on training, nutrition, and health status.

Body fat and lean body mass

Definite benefit

The data reviewed

Data from several randomized controlled studies suggest that lean body mass will very likely increase with testosterone therapy in both elderly and middle-aged/younger men, as well as in men who are eugonadal or hypogonadal.

Lean body mass starts to change at 3 months and can start to plateau at 6 months. Body fat can start to change soon after the lean body mass changes, and begins to plateau at 12–24 months. The changes can extend past that point depending on training, nutrition, and health status.

Figure 5.1

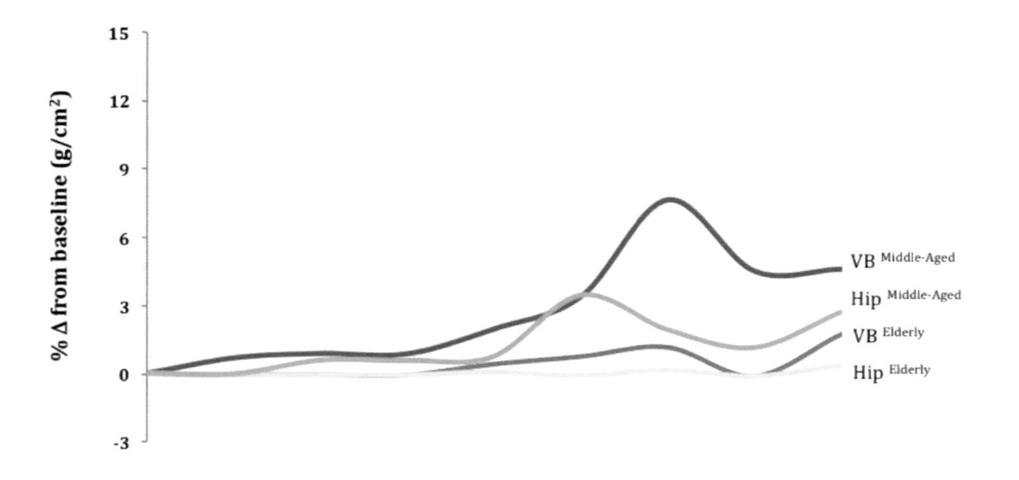

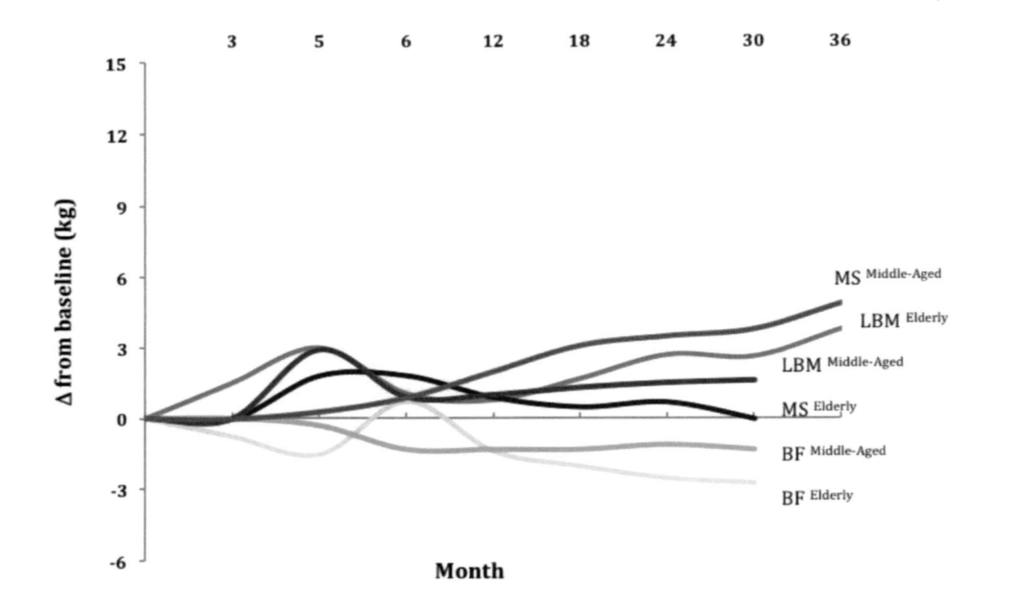

Sexual Domain

Erectile dysfunction and libido

Definite benefit if low testosterone is the cause

The most common sexual complaint consistently associated with testosterone deficiency is decreased libido. ED is also common, but more complex than libido. ED can be a multifactorial diagnosis, the causes of which not only span sexual and emotional domains, but also involve a subset of vascular and neurological physical domain considerations.

ED should prompt investigation into testosterone deficiency and testosterone therapy. Patients with ED of due to problems with circulation might see more robust responses, whereas those with psychological contributions to ED could be less responsive.

In addition to testosterone replacement for men with hypogonadism, daily low-dose phosphodiesterase inhibitors (PDE5) should be considered, such as Cialis. Studies have shown that PDE5 use has benefits beyond ED, including potential improvement in cognition, depression, high blood pressure, and benign enlargement of the prostate.

Improvements in ED begin at 3-6 months, with no further improvement expected after 6 months.

Mood/dysthymia

Probable benefit

There is moderate to strong clinical evidence that aging men with many symptoms related to sense of well-being can benefit from testosterone therapy. Common symptoms in presenting men include depression, cantankerousness, "feeling off their game," less drive, lower motivation, decreased quality of sleep, and decreased ability to concentrate. With treatment, mood begins to improve at 3-6 weeks and starts to plateau at 5-9 months.

Cognition

Possible benefit

Cognitive function is more complex than other domains of testosterone deficiency. However, there are inconsistent reports of improved visuospatial memory for men who optimize their testosterone levels.

Other health parameters that improve with testosterone replacement

- Reduced inflammation. Improvement begins at 3 weeks and peaks around 12 weeks.
- Insulin sensitivity improvess within a few days, but measurable changes in glycated hemoglobin occur at 3–12 months.
- The lipid profile improves at 4 weeks and peaks around 12 months.
- Prostate-specific antigen (PSA) levels can rise marginally, but the effects of testosterone therapy peak at 12 months. Changes after 12 months are not related to testosterone therapy.
- Hematocrit (blood thickness) increases at 3 months and peaks at 12 months.

Summary: Benefits of Testosterone Therapy

Testosterone's efficacy in each domain depends on the dosage, age, severity of deficiency, length of treatment, and other health problems. hormonal/genetic factors (CAG repeat length and estradiol, free fraction estradiol, and cortisol levels) also influence the effectiveness of testosterone treatment.

Physical domain effects are strongly dose dependent., and improvements in the physical domain are strongly dependent on progressive resistance training and nutrition, without which testosterone's impact would likely be substantially limited.

The most consistent effect of testosterone in the physical domain is body fat mass reduction, particularly in terms of visceral fat. The effect on lean body mass follows closely behind the body fat effect. The effect on muscle strength is less consistent, due to a number of factors, such as the FT and TT levels achieved, methodological limitations (study design) and the absence of progressive overload programs.

The effects on BMD are the least consistent, particularly between different age groups, and might be more closely related to the modulation of estradiol, free fraction of estradiol, and IGF-1 levels. Although testosterone's effect is time dependent in all domains, BMD requires the longest time to show effects.

Testosterone's impact on the sexual domain shows discrete thresholds for dose effectiveness. Evidence suggests that younger patients respond more robustly in the physical and sexual domains.

The correction of testosterone deficiency leads to the reversal of these highlighted trends. By correcting low testosterone levels, there is less muscle and bone loss and reduced body fat. Patients who optimize their testosterone levels can expect longer independent living by minimizing their frailty and risk of disability.

HRT Options

Part VI

Introduction

*T*estosterone therapy has been available since testosterone was first isolated and synthesized in the first half of the 20th century. Routes of administration have included nearly the entire gamut. Patients currently enjoy a comprehensive range of options with small clinical differences.

Table 6.1

Timeline of the Emergence of Testosterone Treatments

1931	Isolated A	**1960's**	Synthetics
1935	Isolated T; Synthesized	**1970's**	PO Undecanoate
1940's	Pellets and 17α	**1990's**	Patches
1950's	Esters	**2000's**	Gels

Synthetic testosterones were created in the hope of improving certain aspects of testosterone therapy, such as muscle strength gain. However, synthetic testosterone lacks a complete physiological effect, is unable to convert to DHT or estradiol, and has toxicities not observed with bioidentical testosterone.

Work on synthetic selective testosterone continues, but until its safety has been demonstrated, it is unlikely to appear in clinical practice.

Total serum testosterone levels are not necessarily reflective of testosterone's total biological impact.

The biologic action of testosterone is complex and includes factors that we have already discussed, such as variations in its receptor (the androgen receptor polymorphism). The biologic activity of testosterone is determined in large part by the degree of aromatization of testosterone (i.e., the conversion of testosterone to estradiol). Estradiol, among other factors, is therefore an important marker of the overall biological impact of testosterone, particularly with respect to BMD.

Supplements

No consistent effects have been reported with over-the-counter supplements for testosterone therapy. We therefore cannot recommend supplements such as androstenolone (didehydroepiandrosterone). Focusing on the core program (such as improving nutritional choices and exercise routines and optimizing hormone intake) will yield the best results. Supplements can be an expensive distraction.

Testosterone Therapy Options

There are a variety of methods used to increase testosterone. Each has certain advantages and disadvantages. It is important to note that it is never a matter of one being better than another but rather one being *different* than another. Here again, we see the importance of looking at the individual Needs Analysis. This will determine what method best suits you as an individual. A skilled care provider should be able to use several methods, choosing the one that best fits your specific needs.

General Categories:

1. Direct replacement with testosterone
2. Indirect replacement using clomiphene citrate
3. Indirect replacement using human chorionic gonadotropin (HCG)

Direct administration of testosterone is the most common method of therapy. In cases of primary failure (testicular injury or senescence) it is the only option. In men with secondary failure (low production due to insufficient pituitary signaling) Clomiphene and HCG administration are also options.

Direct replacement with testosterone

There are three categories of direct replacement. Oral, injectable, and transdermal. Injections are most commonly made intramuscularly (IM) but can also be made subcutaneously. Subcutaneous systems include injections and pellet placement. Transdermal systems include sublingual, intranasal, and direct application to the skin with creams, gels, or patches.

All direct forms of testosterone administration lead to full suppression of the hypothalamus, pituitary, and gonadal axis. In other words, it shuts down all natural production and completely takes over the system.

Oral testosterone

Not used

Orally ingested bioidentical testosterone is effectively metabolized (broken down and rendered ineffective) in the liver before it reaches the rest of the body. Therefore, essentially no testosterone action occurs from taking this substance orally.

The oral form must therefore be chemically modified to avoid it being metabolized by the liver, called the "first-pass effect." This modification was first achieved by placing a methyl group in the 17^{α} position of the molecule through an alkylating process. Later, the 17^{β} position was employed to create testosterone undecanoate.

Oral testosterone is not currently in use and has still not been approved in the US for HRT. Early forms of the drug were found to cause liver toxicity.

Transdermal Systems

Transdermal testosterone (direct application to the skin)

Often used

Similar to the sublingual route, the transdermal route avoids the first-pass metabolism by the liver and is therefore more available to the rest of the body. This formulation is often prescribed by care providers. The intra-patient variability in absorption day to day is perhaps the biggest disadvantage to transdermal systems. In addition, direct application to the skin leads to much higher DHT levels, particularly compared with injectables when equivalent serum testosterone levels are reached. Commercial versions are markedly more expensive than injectable forms, although compounded versions reduce some of this difference.

Sexual performance parameters achieved with this form are comparable to other testosterone formulations and routes of administration.

Table 6.2

Advantages and Disadvantages of Transdermal Testosterone

Positives	Negatives
▪ Painless ▪ No peaks and valleys in blood levels ▪ Inexpensive compound versions (not as inexpensive as injectable forms) ▪ Does not cause blood thickening	▪ Requires daily use ▪ Adequate levels can be hard to achieve; less reliable ▪ Gooey consistency ▪ Results in higher DHT levels ▪ Suppresses the pituitary gland

Gels (Androgel)

Often used

Gels are also widely used and provide an alternative to patches. There have been slightly fewer complaints of skin irritation (5.5%) with gels People prefer gels over patches and therefore tend to use them more consistently.

The transfer of testosterone to other people is rare, provided the hands are rinsed and allowed to dry for ten minutes. Hand washing within this time frame does not affect the transfer of testosterone and does not affect absorption.

Patient experience: If contact is anticipated, you should wash the application area after 10 minutes with soap and warm water and cover the skin.

Sublingual

Rarely used

Various forms of sublingual testosterone are available, but we do not find any particular advantage of this route. It avoids the more prominent conversion to DHT seem with application to the skin.

Scrotal patch (Testoderm)

Rarely used

Scrotal skin cells lack a specific enzyme called 5α-reductase inhibitor. This enzyme typically blocks the conversion of testosterone to DHT. A scrotal patch therefore dramatically increases DHT levels. It is not clear whether this is a physiologically adverse event, but high DHT levels are known to increase the risk of hair loss, an undesirable outcome for a large segment of the male population.

Testoderm® was the first transdermal form of testosterone delivery. Skin irritation, difficulty adhering the patch to the skin, and markedly high DHT levels (4- to 10-fold higher than baseline levels) and subsequent hair loss meant that this delivery system was less than optimal and rarely used.

Patient experience: Skin reactions. Possible hair loss from high DHT levels.

Dermal patch (Androderm)

Often used

Dermal patches are widely used and are generally tolerated but tend to cause irritation. Improved tolerance has been shown by placing triamcinolone acetonide 0.1% cream to the patch site before the patch is applied.

Increased hematocrit (thickening of the blood) can persist in 15% of patients after discontinuing the use of patches. The use of patches might result in slightly lower increases in bioavailable testosterone when compared with intramuscular administration, and is therefore less effective.

A return to baseline testosterone levels is achieved within 24 hours, and there is no accumulation. If a patient misses a dose, they might notice adverse effects immediately.

Sexual performance parameters after applying the patches are comparable to those observed with other testosterone formulations and routes of administration.

Patient experience: Skin reactions.

Intranasal

Not frequently used

Intranasal administration of testosterone is available through a gel (Natesto Nasal Gel), which dispenses 5.5 mg/pump. The recommended dosage is 1 pump per nostril 3 times a day, for a total dosage of 33 mg/day.

The disadvantages of this dosing regimen include the number of administrations required each day and the potential for missed doses due to colds. Furthermore, 10% of users will not achieve 300 ng/dL, which is considered a therapeutic dose. Animal models have shown increased intracranial testosterone levels disproportionate to the serum levels. Similar increases can be expected in humans, although the clinical implications are unknown. The bottom line is that the intranasal administration of testosterone is still a new route, one that our practice does not prescribe.

Transdermal testosterone is used more commonly in primary care, does not require an injection, and is therefore painless. The peaks and valleys that occur with the intramuscular route do not occur with transdermal therapy. The degree of blood thickening with transdermal testosterone may be less than that with the injectable administration but this could be due primarily to the fact that peak blood levels generally are not as high as seen with injectables. Both intramuscular and transdermal testosterone therapy suppress the hypothalamus, pituitary gland and testicles.

Transdermal options, however, require daily administration, and adequate testosterone levels can be hard to attain. Drug delivery is less reliable because of daily skin variations, and a greater conversion to DHT occurs due to 5-α-reductase enzymes in the hair follicles.

Injectable testosterone and other methods

Injectable

Often used

Injected testosterone comes in many forms, but typically as esters found in enthanate, cypionate, and undecanoate. Esters are employed to slow the local absorption of testosterone from the muscle into the bloodstream, lowering the water solubility of the steroid and increasing its fat solubility. An ester is a chain composed primarily of carbon and hydrogen atoms. This chain is typically attached to the parent steroid hormone at the 17th carbon position (beta orientation).Generally, the longer the ester chain, the lower the water solubility of the compound and the longer it will take for the full dose to reach general circulation. Esterification provides for less frequent dosing.

Testosterone is therefore altered to avoid the liver's metabolic action. This is achieved by adding an ester to the side of the testosterone, which prevents the liver from metabolizing the testosterone. As the modified testosterone enters the bloodstream from the muscle deposit where it was injected, enzymes in the blood cleave (i.e., chop) off the ester group, leaving testosterone to circulate and perform its action. Due to the fact that the deposit from the muscle injection slowly seeps into the bloodstream and that the enzymes are limited in how quickly they can cleave off the ester, the injected testosterone acts for much longer than other forms of administration.

Testosterone propionate

The typical dosage is 50 mg 2-3 times per week. The drug can be used to improve testosterone therapy, but it is not used as a primary therapy formulation due to the need for frequent injections.

Testosterone enanthate

Typical dosages are 100 mg/week. The testosterone is suspended in sesame oil. It can be thought of as essentially equivalent to testosterone cypionate.

Testosterone cypionate

Often used

The typical dosage is 100 mg/week. It is suspended in cottonseed oil, and is roughly half the cost of enanthate. Older dosing schedules of testosterone were typically 200 mgs every three weeks. The reason for this was the unfounded belief that is was necessary to allow the pituitary gland to recover some function before the next injection. The peak and trough levels seen in this regimen produce markedly suprapysiologic levels, leading to a higher rate of adverse effects. If a lack of suppression at the pituitary level is desired, then one should use clomiphene or HCG, rather than the un-physiologic administration of testosterone by injection.

Testosterone decanoate

Testosterone decanoate is not now used in medical practice, but used to be sold under the name Neotest 250 and could be found in Sustanon 250, a discontinued blend of testosterone esters.

Testosterone undecanoate/Aveed)

Testosterone undecanoate is a long-acting form of injectable testosterone used in Europe which just recently received FDA approval for use in the United States. A long, branched chain ester allows for a dosing frequency of around ten weeks. Because of a rare incidence of pulmonary micro-embolism due possibly to the castor oil used as a carrier, injections must be done by a physician in an approved facility. Currently, the high cost renders the dosing frequency advantage inconsequential over cypionate and enanthate.

Table 6.3

Advantages and Disadvantages of Intramuscular Testosterone

Positives	Negatives
▪ Inexpensive ▪ No refrigeration required ▪ Easy to change dosage ▪ Reliable delivery in men ▪ Does not require daily administration	▪ Requires injection ▪ Peaks and valleys in blood levels ▪ More likely to cause blood thickening ▪ Suppresses the pituitary gland

Intramuscular testosterone is perhaps the least expensive mode of testosterone replacement therapy. Weekly injections are usually sufficient. Using this method, the testosterone is consistently delivered, in contrast to dermal administration.

However, the administration requires an intramuscular injection, which can be disconcerting and involve mild discomfort. With proper instruction, injection is not as limiting a factor as one might think. We instruct our patients to use a 1.0cc Luer Lock syringe and an 18-gauge 1½-inch needle to draw up the testosterone, which easily draws the medication suspended in oil. The large needle bore does not aerosolize the aliquot (i.e., the drawn portion of the testosterone solution is not converted into a fine spray), as would occur with a small gauge needle. We then have the patient switch to a 25-gauge 1-inch needle. Due to the fact that we use a small-bore needle, the Luer Lock syringe is essential, given a moderate amount of pressure is required for the injection. The injection can then be performed in one of the gluteal muscles or the upper outer portion of the vastus lateralis (one of the thigh muscles). Both sites are well tolerated, and the 25-gauge needle minimizes discomfort. As with all testosterone esters, there will be peaks and valleys in the blood levels.

Intramuscular testosterone does cause increased hematocrit readings on laboratory tests. Increased hematocrit is another way of saying that your blood is thicker. The term erythrocytosis is sometimes used to express this condition. This essentially means that your red blood cells are more numerous and that you have more oxygen-carrying capacity, which is usually a positive feature of taking testosterone. In fact, some athletes increase their hematocrit by training at altitude or by taking erythropoietin. The degree of blood thickening that you might experience is related to the length of the polyglutamine repeat segment in the AR (the variation we discussed above). Some men will have minimal increases; however, a subpopulation (5%–7%) of men will experience frank erythrocytosis and will need to lower their blood thickness. Routine blood donation can solve this problem, but you shouldn't wait until your hematocrit is above 53, or you won't be allowed to donate. Such high hematocrit readings will be considered a blood disorder.

As with transdermal therapy, intramuscular testosterone replacement therapy suppresses the entire pituitary system. Within several weeks, secretion of luteinizing hormone (LH) by the pituitary gland will fall to nearly undetectable levels. A certain degree of testicular atrophy induced by LH depression will likely occur over time. The degree of atrophy varies but can be quite substantial in some men. Although this is mostly a cosmetic problem, it can be very important to some individuals. Notwithstanding this very reasonable concern, testosterone therapy is not contraindicated from a medical standpoint by the potential testicular atrophy, due to the therapy's clinical effectiveness and utility.

If you find that intramuscular testosterone is an effective therapy but are concerned about testicular atrophy, a small dose of human chorionic gonadotropin (HCG) can frequently reduce the degree of atrophy.

Effective HCG dosages are usually in the range of 500–750 IU twice a week administered subcutaneously (in the fat under your skin).

Drawbacks of intramuscular testosterone:

- Slightly inconvenient; requires training in the injection procedure
- Castor oil microembolisms have been reported (testosterone undecanoate/Aveed)
- Possibility of significant time outside therapeutic range (especially with short-acting esters)
- Less effective for nonphysical domain symptoms

Injected microspheres

Not frequently used

Our practice does not use injectable microspheres because of the cost and the painful injections. AIT is a viable but expensive option and requires high-volume, relatively painful injections.

Subcutaneous injection

Not frequently used

Testosterone can be administered subcutaneously. This form offers no real advantage over direct intramuscular injection but may be more acceptable to a subset of patients.

Subcutaneous pellet placement

Often used

This method is often used in women and by some practitioners in men. The advantage is the attainment of stable blood levels for a longer period of time (months). However, the dose curve still must be documented for the individual; one cannot simply place the pellets using an arbitrary time frame. Correction of suprapysiologic levels is not possible, and there is a risk of bruising and infection. It requires a minor surgical procedure on the office. The pellet trocar is roughly the diameter of the little finger.

Indirect replacement with human chorionic gonadotropin (HCG)

Human chorionic gonadotropin

Used commonly

Another therapeutic option for low testosterone is HCG. This is particularly effective for low testosterone levels resulting partly from the insufficient secretion of LH (which stimulates the production of testosterone in the testicles) by the pituitary gland. Our practice often uses this therapy in men younger than 50.

The alpha subunit of HCG is identical to the alpha subunit of LH, follicle-stimulating hormone (FSH), and thyroid-stimulating hormone (TSH), though HCG acts more like LH than FSH or TSH. When administered in sufficient doses to men with low testosterone levels due to low pituitary stimulation, HCG is often effective at increasing the testicular production of testosterone.

Men often prefer HCG because it is injected subcutaneously through a very small needle. Thanks to the resulting increase in intra-testicular testosterone production and a small amount of FSH action, the testicles usually do not atrophy to the same degree as seen with testosterone administration, although volume loss does occur. This is because the testicular volume is mainly dependent of the amount of sperm production, and HCG can still reduce sperm counts in some men to a variable degree. As with clomiphene (a drug we will talk about shortly), HCG directly stimulates the testicular production of estrogen (in addition to testosterone). This production can be monitored and addressed without much difficulty.

HCG can be rather expensive when used in very high doses, especially compared with intramuscular testosterone. HCG requires refrigeration and might therefore be less suitable for patients who travel frequently. Given that HCG is a fragile peptide, it can be easily damaged. The vial in which it is reconstituted cannot be shaken or exposed to temperature changes. HCG originally was derived from urinary sources and was therefore a biologic agent, however it is now made from recombinan methods.

HCG is used in the recombinant form (rHCG) rather than in the first-generation urine form (uHCG). HCG is packaged in bottles by compounding pharmacies by prescription. The hormone is provided at various concentrations and injected intramuscularly or subcutaneously twice a week in the mornings. Dosing is made in International Units, with most effective dosing ranging from 500 to 1500 IU twice weekly. Peak production occurs at about 72 hours post injection. Antibody formation is possible, which usually can be overridden by injecting the dose to occupy all antibody sites.

Table 6.4

Advantages and Disadvantages of Human Chorionic Gonadotropin

Positives	Negatives
▪ Stimulates the testicles to produce testosterone ▪ Employs a subcutaneous injection ▪ No testicular atrophy (except at high doses)	▪ Directly stimulates increased estrogen levels ▪ Expensive (especially at high doses) ▪ Requires refrigeration ▪ Can be easily damaged ▪ Is a biologic agent ▪ Suppresses the pituitary gland

Indirect replacement with clomiphene

Clomiphene

Used occasionally

For patients with low testosterone levels due to a lack of pituitary stimulation (low LH), testosterone can be administered directly (intramuscularly). Given that low testosterone levels are not caused by testicular failure, there are other options. If you have low LH levels, clomiphene citrate might also be effective. Clomiphene acts on estrogen receptors, but the net effect is increased testosterone production. This type of drug is known as a selective estrogen receptor modulator (SERM).

Our practice often uses clomiphene in younger men, especially those whose travel does not allow for the use of HCG. The advantages of clomiphene are that it preserves fertility and testicular size. As an oral form, it is easy to use and is reasonably priced, being much less expensive than HCG. However, clomiphene could present challenges similar to those of transdermal therapies in terms of reaching optimal testosterone levels.

Table 6.5

Advantages and Disadvantages of Clomiphene

Positives	Negatives
▪ Oral administration ▪ Reasonable cost ▪ No pituitary gland suppression ▪ Rarely supraphysiological (greater than normally present in the body)	▪ Stimulates estrogen production by the testes ▪ Suppress IGF-1 ▪ Modulates other estrogen receptors (unknown effects) ▪ Might not achieve optimal testosterone levels

Summary: Testosterone Therapy Options

There are several available methods for testosterone replacement therapy. There is considerable debate as to which mode of administration is best, but each has its advantages and disadvantages. Ultimately, however, the mode of administration is not the main issue, an important aspect for you and your care provider to keep in mind.

Based on your symptoms and the laboratory test results, HRT could be warranted. There are reliable means for consistently administering the hormone, providing consistent feedback to care providers and for assessing the hormonal effect.

Unfortunately, the objective measures leave much to be desired. Hormone levels taken from blood and saliva do not reliably reflect the complex factors that result in the net testosterone effect, as we have discussed.

Your care provider needs to consistently and reliably correlate all four of the following: appropriate symptoms, consistent testosterone delivery, consistent feedback, and proper monitoring of the effect. If this cannot be done, you should not be given the hormone.

Your care provider's assessment of the symptoms you report is the best way for assessing how well you will respond to treatment. You should provide this feedback to your care provider.

Target hormone levels, which can be helpful, are always used as a guide. We treat the whole patient and not simply their blood levels. This practice enhances the effectiveness of replacement therapy by going beyond the use of arbitrary numbers either as targets for therapeutic intervention or as thresholds for starting therapy. It is also important to consider that the symptoms of low testosterone levels can overlap considerably with those of other disorders. A knowledgeable clinical assessment can help determine when to initiate therapy and can also serve as a guide for judging the effectiveness of the therapeutic intervention.

For the treatment of primary hypogonadism (low testosterone levels due to testicular injury or age), our only option is to directly administer testosterone. The two most common forms of administration are transdermal and intramuscular injection. As with all forms of therapy, both routes have advantages and disadvantages. The advantage of intramuscular administration, which our practice favors, is the reliable drug delivery, especially in men. When administered intramuscularly, the entire dose is absorbed into the patient's system. The dosage is very easy to adjust, and the drug requires no refrigeration, remaining quite stable at room temperature.

Depending on the clinical setting, most care providers can successfully apply any of these modes of testosterone therapy. Your therapy should be tailored to your needs. If you travel extensively, you might find clomiphene an excellent alternative to HCG. As you progress through your middle years, your responsiveness to HCG could decline, and testosterone therapy might be a more effective approach. There are many ways to increase your testosterone levels. Your care provider can help tailor the approach to fit your needs.

It is important to provide feedback to your care provider, especially during the first few months. Although laboratory levels will be assessed, the important feedback you provide will help direct the treatment program more accurately. At a minimum, your care provider should also measure DHT, estrogen, and pituitary function levels. These compounds interact and need to be monitored along with testosterone. There is considerable individual variation among the hormones and their response to testosterone. Abrupt changes in therapy are not ideal, but trends can be important for you and your care provider to monitor. Your care provider will sometimes add other medications to reduce estrogen or DHT levels, but that should also be based on your specific needs and symptoms. You should find a care provider (and team) that treats you and not your laboratory measurements.

Testosterone therapy is in many ways an ideal therapy. It is very effective at improving a known range of symptoms and has a huge therapeutic window (effective dose versus toxic dose).

The adverse effects of testosterone therapy are mild, easily recognized and easily managed. The therapy is very safe, as we will see in the upcoming sections.

Safety of HRT

Part VII

*T*estosterone therapy is in many ways an ideal therapy. It is very effective at improving a known symptom complex and has a huge therapeutic window (effective dose versus toxic dose). The adverse effects of testosterone therapy are mild, easily recognized and easily managed. The therapy is very safe, as we will see in the upcoming sections.

Introduction

*I*n general, testosterone supplementation is a safe therapeutic option for men with symptoms related to testosterone deficiency.

In this section, we will cover the potential safety issues discussed in the medical literature to help you better understand future headlines on testosterone therapy, which will show up more frequently as the therapy becomes a more popular option for aging men.

The most significant debate between advocates of testosterone therapy and people who take a more restrictive approach revolves around heart disease. The risk of heart disease with testosterone therapy is limited to a minority of patients who already have significant vascular disease or who have rare familial disorders. We therefore strongly recommend an earlier rather than later start to testosterone replacement therapy to minimize such risks.

Appropriate patient selection and monitoring throughout the treatment is essential for minimizing the risk of heart disease, especially for factors affecting thrombosis, inflammation, and blood vessel health.

Younger and leaner patients tend to have better results, with limited risk in terms of prostate disease, increased blood thickness, and heart disease. Patients with obesity are more likely to experience adverse vascular effects, unless the testosterone therapy is an adjunct to sustained body fat reduction.

The healthier you are when you start testosterone therapy, the more likely the therapy will be safe (and effective) for a long period of time.

Testosterone therapy could be warranted for patients with obesity to assess its added benefit to a sound exercise and nutritional program aimed at reducing body fat and improving function but not as a weight loss agent.

Although not current standard practice, screening patients for heart disease is warranted. Ideally, we should screen for overall blood vessel health; however, the technology for this screening is not yet fully developed. Screening can include physical stress testing, laboratory tests, and imaging studies to determine a baseline cardiovascular risk profile. The baseline profile will assist the decision making when weighing the potential risks of testosterone therapy.

Before we dive into the reported risks of testosterone therapy, we will review how testosterone therapy has been shown to reduce premature death in men. After all, you have to balance the risk with the benefits. Although some risks sound ominous, they need to be understood in terms of real risk, rather than relative risk. We use death (mortality) as an end marker for all benefits and find it useful without necessarily breaking down each of the benefits we discussed in the previous chapters.

Think of mortality as the sum of all risks and benefits. If you live longer than other people similar to you who did not take testosterone, the net balance of risk versus benefit leans more towards the benefit side.

Men with Testosterone Deficiency Die Earlier

Low testosterone and increased mortality

Low testosterone levels are associated with an increased mortality risk in both young and elderly patients, a fact well established in the medical literature.

Studies of young men with untreated hypogonadism (those with a lifelong deficiency) have shown increased mortality rates.

Studies of elderly men with hypogonadism have shown increased all-cause mortality rates with hypogonadal conditions, with data suggesting that the increased rate is due to heart and respiratory disease. A 12-year study of elderly men showed a 40% increase in the mortality rate for patients who were in the lowest quartile for testosterone levels (total and free testosterone), regardless of lifestyle, age, and body fat.

Based on the literature, testosterone deficiency is an independent risk factor for premature death, regardless of known associated health conditions such as obesity and type II diabetes mellitus (DMII).

Heart Disease

Recent studies relating testosterone therapy to increased heart disease risk

Elderly men can be at risk because they might have established heart disease.

The current studies have many flaws, which are similar to those of the Women's Health Initiative (WHI) study of HRT in women.

HRT in men with low testosterone levels has been shown to reduce mortality by approximately 50%, when compared with controls who did not undergo replacement therapy. The reduction in mortality was observed in healthy men but not in those with pre-existing heart disease. These data support our knowledge of the window of opportunity for treating men with HRT.

Despite the reduction in mortality rates, not all studies have concluded that testosterone therapy improves heart disease risk factors, implying that testosterone use is a potential source of increased risk of cardiovascular-related death. Three studies, in particular, are worth examining in detail.

An increased number of adverse events were reported during the Testosterone in Older Men study, a small, randomized controlled study that employed testosterone gel and assessed the adverse outcomes for elderly men (similar to the WHI trial with women). The high number of adverse outcomes resulted in the early termination of the study. A careful examination of the data from that study, however, reveals that the adverse events associated with testosterone administration (categorized according to the Medical Dictionary for Regulatory Activities) included a broad range of events, from peripheral swelling in the legs, high blood pressure and electrocardiogram changes to cardiac events such as heart attacks and stroke.

However, the authors also noted that there was no significant difference in serious adverse events between those who were supplemented with testosterone and those who were not.

The authors also cautioned against drawing broad conclusions about testosterone safety from the study due to the trial's small sample size and its focus on an elderly population. In short, if you are not elderly, the data do not apply to you. If you are elderly, the risk of serious adverse events is not increased, according to the authors who wrote the article.

Another study worth noting is a Veterans Administration (VA) population-based study published in *JAMA* in 2013, which concluded that testosterone therapy in men (average age of 60.6 years) with low testosterone levels is a risk factor for adverse events (i.e., the therapy is not cardioprotective). All of the men underwent coronary angiography during the study.

The study's VA patient population had significant pre-existing blood vessel and heart-related diseases: 90% had high blood pressure, 54.8% had documented obstruction of heart arteries, 53.2% had DMII,

19.5% had peripheral vascular disease (in the legs), 20.3% had had a prior heart attack and 11.1% had had a prior stroke. It is therefore no surprise that a number of the patients experienced further heart disease-related events.

The VA study had an average duration of testosterone therapy of 376 days (a little over a year during the 6-year course of the investigation). Topical dosing was employed by 65% of the patients (gel and patches). Topical preparations have a higher conversion to DHT than injections, which could have unknown risks for heart disease.

The strong conclusions made by the VA study are questionable, given the short period of time and the low doses employed. However, if the conclusions were correct, the adverse effects would likely have shown up far earlier in the longer-term studies and in those that employed more consistent doses of testosterone. In contrast, several better-designed, randomized controlled studies have shown that testosterone therapy improves a number of intermediate outcomes and heart disease risk factors.

The questions raised by the VA study data should not, however, be dismissed entirely. There are physiological mechanisms that could reasonably explain a propensity toward thrombosis with testosterone therapy, as described in the Efficacy section.

> ***It is important to note that younger middle-aged men without heart disease showed no increased risk of heart attack, suggesting a window of opportunity for treating men with low testosterone levels.***

A population cohort study (with patients enrolled in the Truven Health MarketScan database from around the US) showed that the primary outcome of nonfatal acute myocardial infarction was increased in older men and in younger men *with pre-existing heart disease*. The data from this study indicate several notable trends, which are supported by other studies. First, elderly treated men had a substantially increased risk of heart disease events, approximately 3 times the risk when compared with younger men. The risk of heart disease events increased with age in all categories. In contrast, the younger men (<55 years) showed no increased risk or even a small reduced risk. In fact, the only patients younger than 65 with increased risk were those with a prior history of heart disease, as reflected by their relative risk of 1.90.

> ***The Truven study provides interesting data suggesting that the potential increase in heart disease risk with testosterone therapy is probably not the result of increased sexual and physical activity.***

Patients prescribed phosphodiesterase inhibitors (Viagra) did not experience an increased risk of myocardial infarction.

The above studies show a correlation (association) between testosterone use and increased heart disease. A cause and effect relationship for increased heart disease events in patients with *pre-existing blood vessel and heart disease* might eventually be found.

Plausible molecular explanations for this association include increased blood thickness (hematocrit) with the pro-inflammatory effects of testosterone regulated through increased thromboxane A_2 and vascular cell adhesion molecule 1 (VCAM-1) levels.

Summary: Heart Disease

As our experience with the WHI data analysis has shown, aging patients with established atherosclerotic disease are at risk from sex-specific HRT. Treating men for testosterone deficiency might therefore be protective at earlier ages but place them at risk if begun in later years. Although a specific threshold age has not been established, we believe that patients 35–45 years of age are at the lowest risk. Due to the lack of established threshold ages in the literature, various types of exercise, and laboratory and imaging studies might be offered by your care providers to fully assess your heart disease risk.

Patient selection is critical in determining any treatment, particularly one with such a broad impact as testosterone therapy. As Hak et al demonstrated, the detrimental effects of low testosterone levels regardless of cardiac risk factors, indicate that low testosterone levels have an independent effect on heart disease.

Future randomized controlled studies need to be tailored to younger (age 35–45), healthier patients and include specific heart disease endpoints rather than widely separated endpoints that might be statistically but not clinically significant.

Laboratory data that include DHT and estradiol levels might be critical for determining who is at risk, as would their inflammation and coagulation markers. Testosterone-related markers (such as thromboxane A_2 and VCAM-1) and estrogen-related markers (such as activated protein C resistance and decreased coagulation inhibitors) should be considered in future studies. These factors might be important for determining the proper patient populations and monitoring requirements for testosterone therapy for minimizing heart disease risk.

For men with risk factors for heart disease, the risks of testosterone therapy might outweigh the benefits.

A common factor in all of the studies mentioned above is that none of them would be described as using state-of-the-art therapy. Several of the studies approached HRT for men in a rather ham-fisted manner, with poor follow up, lack of monitoring, nonexistent treatment targets and lack of management for DHT and estradiol levels. It is therefore not surprising that the results were mixed at best.

We believe that properly managed testosterone therapy has little heart disease risk and great potential benefit. Although it might be prudent to use a different approach for patients with known heart disease or advanced age (through slower progression to treatment levels, more aggressive management of adverse effects, etc.), we believe that neither factor is a contraindication for replacement therapy.

In our practice, we assess the heart disease and metabolic risk of all of our patients, reviewing the family history and blood work. We employ dual energy X-ray absorptiometry (DXA) to measure BMD, carotid ultrasounds, VO_2 (maximal oxygen consumption) testing and physical examinations. Finally, we prescribe therapy based upon the individual needs analysis.

Testosterone improves the health of healthy vessels but increases the risk for diseased vessels.

How can testosterone be attributed to increased heart disease, while a deficit of testosterone is simultaneously attributed to heart disease?

Based on our more than 15 years of clinical experience and a detailed review of the current medical literature, we believe that testosterone replacement therapy is safe when properly administered to appropriate patients. The *LG Window of Opportunity* accounts for the paradoxical effects of testosterone therapy on heart disease.

> ***Patients who have a substantial burden of pre-existing heart disease when starting testosterone therapy might be at risk.***

Care providers can help assess whether or not you have such a burden. A comprehensive assessment of your heart health is part of our practice's standard workup for all patients. Your heart disease risk can be determined from your family history, an assessment of your cholesterol levels (using cutting-edge cholesterol markers, if necessary), a measurement of your carotid artery wall thickness (carotid intima media thickness) and a measurement of VO_2 max through exercise testing. If you have multiple risk factors for heart disease, we can conduct further studies that directly examine your heart vessels (64-slice CT angiography or direct heart artery catheterization) and can tell us more about your risk for testosterone therapy. In the near future, we expect even better tests for measuring your heart health and the general condition of your blood vessels.

Men with documented heart disease who are optimally managed can be safely treated with a closely monitored conservative approach to replacement therapy. Lower doses, more aggressive blood donations (to prevent the blood from getting too thick) and aspirin (antiplatelet therapy) can further reduce the risk in higher risk patients.

Preventive measures can minimize heart disease risk and should be the hallmark of the care provider's approach, specifically if you already have documented risk of heart disease.

We believe that the above measures are the missing pieces of the puzzle regarding most current approaches to the treatment of testosterone deficiency.

As with prostate cancer and testosterone therapy, there appears to be a paradoxical relationship between heart disease and testosterone therapy. On one hand, it is well documented that mortality due to heart disease is nearly 2:1 for men versus women, which suggests that testosterone (the male sex hormone) is an independent risk factor for heart disease. On the other hand, evidence tells us that testosterone deficiency is strongly associated with heart disease. Hence, the paradox: How can testosterone be attributed to increased heart disease while a deficiency of testosterone is simultaneously associated with higher rates of heart disease?

A U-shaped curve relating testosterone levels to mortality could theoretically exist. We see this relationship with growth hormone and IGF-1 (a marker of growth hormone). A U-shaped curve means that mortality rates (on the y axis) are higher when testosterone levels (on the X axis) are either too high or too low. There might be various mechanisms at play at the high and low levels. We do not know if this is definitely the case for testosterone as it is for growth hormone because the vast majority of studies have only examined individuals at low and low-normal levels of testosterone. Most studies do not analyze large groups of patients in the upper ranges of normal.

If there is a U-shaped relationship between mortality and testosterone levels, it might be due to other disease conditions, such as pre-existing heart disease and DMII. These conditions could shift the balance of testosterone effects on the blood vessel lining (endothelium) creating a pro-inflammatory state (which can increase the risk of clogged vessels, heart disease, and strokes).

LG Window of Opportunity Hypothesis for HRT in Aging Patients

It has been conclusively shown that women are at greater risk of heart disease when undergoing estrogen replacement if more than 10 years have elapsed since menopause. During this period, the "risk gap" for atherosclerosis and heart disease between men and women narrows. This finding suggests that estrogen and/or progesterone are cardioprotective prior to the onset of menopause. If estrogen is administered before atherosclerotic disease evolves during the critical window period, the increased heart disease risk is neutralized, and the benefits of estrogen for heart disease outweigh the risks. If estrogen is administered to postmenopausal women after the critical window has closed, their risk of embolic events via plaque destabilization increases. A similar mechanism might exist for testosterone therapy in men.

- Men with established (but not necessarily documented) heart disease might be at risk from testosterone therapy, whereas men with no such disease might benefit from the positive effects of testosterone through increased flow-mediated dilation, the anti-inflammatory characteristics of testosterone and improved lipid profile and fat metabolism. Treatment during the window of opportunity when blood vessel health is optimal will result in the most benefit and the least risk. The net effect of testosterone is mixed but usually emerges as a net positive effect in young healthy patients. This delicate balance of effects can be more easily tipped toward a net negative effect with testosterone therapy in patients with a diseased vascular state.

The safe treatment of men with testosterone therapy could therefore involve a narrower window than the treatment of women with HRT. Randomized controlled studies that compare healthy middle-aged men to elderly men, with reliable documentation of the atherosclerotic disease burden, could help establish the cardiovascular safety of testosterone therapy.

Other Heart Diseases

Systolic/diastolic blood pressure and heart rate changes

Improved heart rates and blood pressure using testosterone therapy have been reported in the literature. In clinical practice, however, we have not observed a noticeable change in blood pressure or baseline heart rates with testosterone therapy alone. Exercise and nutrition are more likely to have a substantial impact on these parameters.

Changes in the cholesterol profile

A general shift toward a favorable lipid profile is often observed in patients, except those with a high BMI. The benefits of high HDL-C (the "good" cholesterol) levels are commonly *not* seen in patients with high BMI.

LDL-C (the "bad" cholesterol) levels are generally reduced in most patients. HDL-C levels can initially decrease marginally, especially in patients who achieve testosterone levels in the upper quartile. However, this imbalance is effectively neutralized or even reversed with aggressive nutrition and exercise programs. Thus, in our practice, net HDL-C levels often tend toward a more favorable profile (high).

Prostate Disease

Prostate Cancer Statistics

Prostate cancer is the third leading cause of cancer-related deaths among men in Western countries, preceded only by lung and colon cancer. The most substantial risk factors are age, family history and ethnicity.

The prevalence of prostate cancer varies by country, with Canada and the US having the highest global prevalence. The following statistics published by the National Cancer Institute refer to 2013 data for the US.

Table 7.1

Prostate Cancer Statistics

New Cases	238,590 (a slow downward trend)
Deaths	29720 (3rd highest cancer mortality)
5-year survival rate	99.2% (an upward trend)
% of all new cancers	14.4%
% of all cancer deaths	1%
Prevalence	1.7%

Adapted from Siegel et al.

The risk myth: Prostate cancer

Testosterone therapy does not increase the risk of prostate cancer

The impact of testosterone on benign prostatic hypertrophy (an enlarged prostate)

As predicted by the saturation model (discussed below), the effect of TT on prostate gland growth is most notable in patients who have markedly low baseline testosterone levels.

> ***Enlargement of the prostate gland does not occur in men who have normal testosterone levels.***

This is probably due to a volume recovery process that occurs when the previously testosterone-deprived prostate gland responds to normal levels of testosterone. In essence, patients with low testosterone levels likely have small prostates that grow to normal size as the levels return to normal. Once a normal size has been re-established, the prostate gland grows no further. This hypothesis is supported by the fact that men with benign prostatic hypertrophy do not show worse symptoms when starting testosterone therapy.

The myth of prostate cancer and the saturation model

Prostate cancer rates are not higher in aging men with normal testosterone levels.

Initial reports that testosterone levels were directly associated with prostate cancer were misleading and largely based on a single case report. A similar misunderstanding of the literature occurred with saturated fats, which were initially blamed for heart disease (a myth we discussed in the *Nutrition* chapter). The authors of the initial reports that associated higher testosterone levels with higher rates of prostate cancer proposed this cause-and-effect relationship because their data indicated that lowering TT levels leads to the regression of advanced prostate cancer, a finding that has since been confirmed by other researchers. Case reports in 1997 and 1999 also supported the belief that prostate cancer is caused by increased total testosterone levels. The erroneous conclusion drawn by the general medical community from these reported cases was that high testosterone levels lead to prostate cancer.

Marks et al. investigated the saturation model at a cellular level. They found that testosterone supplementation increases DHT and total testosterone levels in the prostate glands of men with hypogonadism. However, when the authors administered testosterone to eugonadal men, there was no statistical increase in DHT and total testosterone levels within the prostate gland. Therefore, when men who have normal testosterone levels are administered testosterone, their prostate glands show no increase in testosterone or metabolite (e.g., DHT) levels. This finding suggests that men who have low testosterone levels (and not those with normal levels) are at risk for prostate cancer progression.

The real risk of prostate cancer and testosterone therapy

The risk of prostate cancer for men undergoing HRT is usually the same or lower than that of men not undergoing HRT.

There is strong evidence that prostate cancer is less likely to occur in men whose testosterone levels are comparable to those of young men with normal levels. This conclusion is also supported by clinical experience. Men's testosterone levels are highest during their early twenties, although prostate cancer is exceedingly rare at this age.

> ***If high testosterone levels cause prostate cancer, we would see a much higher incidence of prostate cancer among young patients.***

In contrast, elderly men have lower testosterone levels and are the ones at risk for prostate cancer. This statement is also supported in the literature. There is strong evidence suggesting that lower testosterone levels are a risk factor for prostate cancer and for prostate cancer with more aggressive characteristics. Nearly half a million men have been assessed in longitudinal studies, which have shown no association between increased testosterone and increased prostate cancer. In fact, prostate cancer rates have been shown to be twice as high among patients with total testosterone levels in the lowest third.

In short, evidence shows that *the risk of prostate cancer in a patient undergoing testosterone therapy is equal to or less than that of the general population*, with one caveat: patients with a history of prostate cancer treated with androgen deprivation are at increased risk for recurrence. Ironically, this specific condition occurred in the original study that raised the generalized, misdirected fear of prostate cancer risk in patients undergoing testosterone therapy.

Testosterone after prostatectomy with androgen deprivation therapy

Testosterone therapy is absolutely contraindicated for patients who have undergone androgen deprivation therapy for prostate cancer.

Testosterone after prostatectomy without androgen deprivation therapy

Generally, if you have had prostate cancer, it is best to avoid testosterone therapy.

Standards of care and common sense suggest that it is prudent to avoid administering testosterone therapy to any patient with a hormone sensitive malignancy, regardless of treatment. Data on such patients in the medical literature is scarce and mixed.

A highly motivated and informed patient, however, might be willing to assume the risk of recurrence, however high, in order to ameliorate the numerous symptoms that are treatable with testosterone therapy.

Until we have larger, randomized controlled studies, we will not be able to properly guide patients on the specific level of risk involved.

Screening recommendations for prostate cancer

PSA levels and digital rectal examinations (DREs) are required before applying testosterone therapy.

Prostate cancer screening recommendations, as with those for testosterone therapy, vary considerably and are based on limited data.

The American Urological Association recommends annual PSA testing and DREs beginning at 50 years of age, with PSA levels >4 ng/mL as the cutoff for diagnostic biopsy evaluations. The American Cancer Society has the same recommendations.

Comments on digital rectal exam

DREs are required for complete physical examinations before applying testosterone therapy.

Data suggest that DREs are of little value for detecting prostate cancer, but clinical observations have demonstrated that some high-grade cancers can be detected before PSA levels have risen significantly. Therefore, it is worth offering DRE in addition to testing PSA levels and letting the patient choose.

Erythrocytosis (Increased Blood Thickening)

Most men will experience blood thickening with HRT. If the thickness rises above normal, blood can be donated to reduce the thickening.

Erythropoiesis (blood thickening)

Hematocrit is a laboratory reading to measure how many blood cells are in the bloodstream. If the hematocrit is too low, the patient is in an anemic state. Anemia can be associated with generalized weakness and ineffective tissue oxygenation because there are insufficient red blood cells to carry the oxygen to the tissues. Many chronic illnesses are associated with anemia, and many men who have low testosterone levels are mildly anemic.

> ***Typically, testosterone therapy results in a 3- to 4-point increase in hematocrit. This often brings patients with mild anemia into the normal range, one of the positive effects of testosterone therapy.***

Occasionally, patients will respond more vigorously to testosterone therapy, and their hematocrit will rise above the normal range. This condition is sometimes called polycythemia, but the more correct term is erythrocytosis, given that the levels of other blood components (such as white blood cells and platelets) do not rise with testosterone. The net result is a theoretically higher probability of blood coagulating (forming clots) due to the increased viscosity of the blood. Clots in the arteries can cause heart attacks and strokes. Clots in the veins can cause pulmonary emboli (clots that block lung vessels from getting oxygen). The risk of clots is easy to minimize by periodically monitoring the hematocrit levels and donating blood when the levels reach approximately 52. Low-dose aspirin (81 mg) is recommended for most patients over the age of 40. You can ask your care provider whether aspirin is a good choice for you.

Effects on hematocrit levels are evident at 3 months and peak at 9–12 months.

Venous Thromboembolism

Testosterone therapy can uncover a genetic predisposition to blood clots.

As we discussed above, it is well known that testosterone therapy results in a rise of hematocrit, such that therapeutic blood donations might be required for safety reasons.

The risk of clots is also related to other factors, in addition to the hematocrit level. A number of studies have suggested that testosterone therapy can uncover a predisposition to clots from inherited coagulation defects. Most of these rare events have been reported within 1 year of the testosterone therapy. To date, none of the events have contributed to death. A careful family history review is recommended to increase awareness of the presence of a clotting disorder that might be uncovered during testosterone therapy. The prevalence of these problems is approximately 1%.

Summary: Safety of HRT for Men

The safety of testosterone therapy is an ongoing concern, and studies with sufficient power are required to establish definitive guidelines. Current data strongly support the safety of testosterone therapy in men with no documented prostate disease, normal PSA levels and normal digital rectal examinations.

> ***Overall death rates indicate that men with low testosterone levels who participate in testosterone therapy have lower (as much as 50% lower) death rates when compared with untreated men.***

Heart disease is an area of strong interest due to the conflicting onclusions in recent population studies. Although there are problems vith these studies in terms of competency of administration and nonitoring, there are plausible mechanisms by which testosterone ould cause problems in *a subgroup of men with pre-existing substantial ardiac plaque burden* (e.g., those with increased blood thickness). n addition, increased estrogen levels (by conversion from high stosterone levels) could increase blood clotting complications due to e effects of estrogen on the liver. It seems prudent to be more cautious hen applying the therapy to men suspected of having substantial heart isease burden. Frequent monitoring and more aggressive management f blood thickening (through blood donations) and anti-platelet therapy (aspirin) could help reduce some of the risk for this group of men. The presence of heart disease should not be a direct contraindication for testosterone replacement therapy. In our experience, this risk has been low. It should be noted that our practice focuses strongly on lifestyle management, which substantially reduces the risk of myocardial infarction, regardless of testosterone therapy.

Additional research to corroborate the result of the initial studies would be invaluable in verifying this reduced mortality.

Contraindications Part VIII

Introduction

*T*here are few absolute contraindications to testosterone therapy. As with all medicine, careful consideration needs to be given the entire clinical setting before implementing a therapy.

Absolute

Prostate cancer and breast cancer (in men) are absolute contraindications for testosterone therapy. Therefore, DREs, PSA measurements and breast examinations are required for all patients prior to testosterone therapy. Prolactin levels are also recommended.

There is universal agreement that testosterone therapy is contraindicated for patients with prostate cancer, especially those treated with androgen deprivation therapy. In the future, we will hopefully have consensus regarding heart disease as a possible relative contraindication for testosterone therapy. If you are predisposed to blood clots and have liver disease, obstructive sleep apnea or congestive heart failure, the benefits of testosterone replacement therapy should be carefully weighed against the risk of exacerbating these conditions.

Conclusion

Part IX

Despite decades of research on the relationship between testosterone and its impact on the physical, sexual and emotional domains of men, the issue of who benefits most from testosterone therapy is still under consideration.

The literature is replete with data confirming that men with low testosterone levels have higher rates of other diseases (e.g., heart disease) and higher mortality. It is less obvious who benefits the most and in what way.

There is mixed evidence regarding the correlation between the benefits and the testosterone levels. Evidence suggests that men with extremely low testosterone levels could benefit more substantially than those with less severe deficiencies, but often the duration of the deficiency is a bigger concern for optimizing the response. Long-term testosterone deficiency could desensitize patients to the effects of circulating testosterone.

> ***A delay in the diagnosis of testosterone deficiency could be a significant issue in determining your responsiveness to testosterone therapy.***

The dosage and duration of testosterone therapy are also variables to consider when determining the optimal clinical treatment. In differing circumstances, the dosage and duration of the testosterone therapy can be quite varied. For example, achieving muscle mass gain in a pre-frail or younger patient at risk for frailty might require only periodic use of testosterone therapy. Lower dosages to threshold levels, in contrast, could be the minimum required to address ED.

Younger men with low testosterone levels are consistently the greatest beneficiaries of testosterone therapy, particularly when testosterone deficiency is diagnosed early and is an isolated condition, rather than part of a syndrome.

With advancing age, other diseases (such as heart disease) could play an additive role in reducing the efficacy of testosterone therapy, partly because testosterone deficiency is only one factor contributing to the syndrome and in part because of the direct contradictory effects of other diseases (especially inflammation).

Elderly men have shown mixed responsiveness in the physical, sexual, and cognitive domains. The most consistent responses have been seen in the sexual domain, at threshold levels below 8 nmol/L (231 ng/dL) for erections and 12 nmol/l (346 ng/dL) for libido. In the physical domain, elderly patients most often experience limited but significant reductions in body fat. In particular, these patients experience reduced visceral fat, which is most closely associated with earlier death. However, the remaining parameters in the physical domain, such as BMD and muscle strength, have shown inconsistent results.

The mixed responses by elderly men in these elements of the physical domain are likely due to several factors. The authors of most studies in this field have employed flawed methods for training and assessing muscle strength. None of the studies by these authors included a control with a specific exercise program. Many studies simply forbade exercise in order to remove it as a factor. Participating in testosterone therapy without exercise, however, is not going to yield gains in strength. It is therefore unclear what the authors hoped to accomplish by not allowing their patients to exercise. Despite this, the endpoints of most of these studies involved the assessment of strength gains. Many of these studie tested strength using isometric or isokinetic methods, which are rarel used in strength training. Most people who spend time in the gym trai with isotonic methods (free weights and weight-training machines). Thus, although the testing methodology itself is reproducible, it is not a valid assessment of the training undertaken by the patients. In addition, the mixed strength results in elderly patients are likely due to a general age-related blunting of exercise response. In particular, the blunted response is affected by pro-inflammatory agents such as interleukin 6. Inconsistent results in BMD are partly due to the fact that many of the studies were short. BMD, however, can take 1–2 years to increase. BMD also depends largely on the known process of converting testosterone to estradiol. Everyone's body does this to varying degrees of efficiency. Changes in BMD are therefore likely to vary considerably from individual to individual.

Brain health (cognitive domains) in the elderly requires complicated assessments. Testing methods are highly variable, although they are usually performed with "validated" methods. At least 8 separate areas of brain health are regularly tested, but only one of these areas (the visual/spatial memory) shows mildly consistent improvement with testosterone therapy in the elderly. The improvement of scores could be due in part to increased speed of recognition rather than improved accuracy.

Middle-aged men (45–65 years of age) with low testosterone levels have been the least studied of the three age groups. However, the few studies that have been performed in the context of broader investigations strongly suggest that testosterone-deficient but otherwise healthy middle-aged men might be excellent candidates for testosterone therapy.

In particular, the all-cause mortality rates study by Shores et al. showed a reduced mortality rate of 50% in middle-aged men treated with testosterone therapy, compared with the control groups.

In contrast, a study by Basaria et al. of 209 elderly patients was erminated early due to significantly increased cardiovascular events in e treated group. Most of the men in these studies had highly variable oses and duration of testosterone therapy and often had significant eart disease risk factors before starting treatment. Nevertheless, our experience of women with HRT through the WHI study warrants the full consideration of the possibility that treating men in early middle age, before significant heart disease has been established, could be the optimal time for implementing testosterone therapy. Treating men later could place them at significant risk for heart disease and strokes.

Future studies on testosterone therapy should be designed with the goal of determining the population that the therapy benefits, the optimal time and the optimal dosage for the therapy.

We are currently working under the hypothesis of the *LG Window of Opportunity* for HRT and believe that thorough testing for heart disease and the early treatment of low testosterone levels will optimize both the benefit and safety of testosterone therapy.

Made in the USA
Las Vegas, NV
28 December 2023

83593254R00197